LAURA NAUDIN
Testimony

A cancer and thousand needles

Why this book?

At 10 years old, having read «Anne Frank's Diary» ever since, I have never stopped writing in my diary with the secret hope of one day being published too ... without the tragic end!
In college, my French teacher, Ms. Haida, evolved my taste for writing and I created a blog that I continue to maintain today.

I am fortunate to have my four grandparents, this book is primarily intended for them. So some details might seem trivial, but I have to tell you that I refrained from explaining what Instagram is.

Perhaps it will be of use to all those who are going through the ordeal of cancer and who can recognize themselves or those around them who do not always know how to react.

With the transcription of my diary, I want to free myself from the burden of the disease and lift the taboo so that you dare to talk about cancer.

Because I don't want to erase anything, I don't want to forget anything, this is my story.

Thanks

Thanks to my boyfriend, Flavien,
to my parents, Valérie and Pascal,
to my in-laws, Laurence and Patrick,
for their patience, their listening
and the help I needed.

Thanks to the onco-hemato team
from the Bretonneau hospital in Tours.

Thanks to my Irish family
for whom I did this rough translation.

From yarn to needle

French expression who mean : one thing led to another

January 2018,

- What is breakdown? A big depression? Well, I definitely have that.

Me, the hyperactive, don't want anything anymore. My fixed-term contract has just ended and I spend my days on the sofa. I am fed up with everything. It's because of this apartment ! It's cold there, it's too small for two. And while I'm glad that my boyfriend, Flavien, is more and more at home, after seven months of dating, I feel like it is choking me. I'm used to live alone.

I need to take care of these itchy patches on my face and neck. They appeared in August 2017, just after the operation on my heel. We thought the lump in my bone was cancerous ... But no, it was some kind of cyst. My heel looked like an empty shell, so very fragile. The «hole» was filled with biomaterials and bone from my pelvis. Months of crutches followed.

For my itching, I saw a first dermatologist who hesitated between psoriasis and eczema, she prescribed me strong drug that I refused. The second explains to me that this will be settled with the arrival of sunny days, because my skin lacks sunlight and he suggests his UV cabin. Not at all convinced, I would like a third opinion, I turned to the dermatology department at the Tours hospital, where an intern prescribed me new creams. But after these three inconclusive opinions and a dozen more or less soft and healthy creams, I am looking for alternative solutions to get rid of my plaques and take advantage of them to be less stressed. So I try to go see a magnetizer, I try meditation applications and shiatsu. Nothing I tried remove my plaques.

For my foot, I have had physiotherapy sessions every week since December and each time it hurts somewhere or I'm not in good shape. I confide in my physiotherapist and apologize, because it's not my habit.

10 p.m. one evening in March, a strong pain in my chest. My heart ? My lungs ? I am not the type to worry so I decline the proposal of my boyfriend who wants the intervention of S.O.S doctor.

- It only lasted a few seconds! Nothing to be alarmed about. But I'm exhausted, I'm going to bed.

I make an appointment with my doctor. I explain to hem that at the moment I'm not in good shape, I think I'm depressed. Nothing to report during auscultation. She thinks of a rejection of my heel bone graft. As I have a check-up in April, in orthopedics, with the professor who operated me, I will do a full check-up. To prove that there is nothing nowhere and that the problem is with my heel. Blood test, urine test and an x-ray of the lungs which she advises me to do in the private clinic next to my house, to go faster.

A few days later, we are in Bordeaux for the Bigflo and Oli concert, my birthday present from Flavien for my 24th birthday. The day before, I feel this chest pain again, followed by a great discomfort. I promise Flavien to take my blood test when I get home, I've been dragging my feet for a week to get to the laboratory.

Blood test done! Two days later, my doctor's replacement called me a little distraught.

- Miss, are you feeling well? Can you stand up and do your activities?
- Yes, I'm fine, I'm in good shape.

My white blood cell count has exploded, there's an infection somewhere. I'm not warning, it's certainly my foot, but it bothers me if I have to repeat the operation on that damn heel or ... maybe it's another patient's toll.

On my X-ray the following week, the radiologist asks me if I'm coughing. Indeed, I have been coughing for several weeks like a cold that will not come out, nothing surprising at the beginning of spring. I go into the ultrasound room to examine my entire chest and stomach. After the exams, the doctor at the clinic explained to me that he saw an eleven centimeter mass in my left lung and that it could be pneumonia. He prescribed a scanner and I left with my radio under my arm. I decide to make an appointment in the public hospital, where I was treated for my foot. The scanner is expected in a month, mid-May.

In the meantime, I have an appointment with the Professor for the third check of my heel. My foot is fine, but he considers my chest x-ray to be worrying and the time to take the scan far too long. He calls the imaging department.

- What do you have available before the end of the week?

It's Monday, he manages to get me a time slot for Friday, twenty days ahead of schedule. He also explains to me that for older people, after a transplant like I had a chest x-ray is always done. We might have seen this mass earlier.

I feel weaker and weaker, I can't stand my straining bra anymore, my shoulder hurts, I don't know what's going on in my body, but something is wrong not. Mum decides to take me to the emergency room. A mad world patient in the room, I can hardly stand up. The intern makes us come quickly.

- If you come for a scan earlier, you can go home or you can wait 6-10 hours, but nothing more will be done.

Despite his virulent speech, I decide to wait, because I'm really not in good shape and I don't understand why. After two hours, I am taken care of. The doctor takes my case more seriously. Blood test, new X-ray... Arrive in the evening, the doctor suggests that I stay or come back tomorrow for a Doppler in order to check if my arteries are not blocked. I live next door, I choose to go back and sleep in my bed. I'm not resting very well at the moment so Flavien is sleeping on the sofa. He wants to stay by my side and hardly ever comes home to his parents.

The next day, an icy welcome from the radiologist who will perform my Doppler. He doesn't understand the value of the exam and grumbles that it won't help, that he won't find anything. After a few minutes of pressing hard on my neck, his face changes, he does not look at me and goes to look for a colleague. He saw a mass behind my collarbone. Together they count and they measure without explaining to me, I understand that other masses are visible. I get dressed and laugh to hide my annoyance.

- You see, finally, I didn't come here for nothing!

They just tell me to wait for the scanner to know the nature of the masses.

Friday 27th of April, I go to the scanner while Flavien takes his TOEIC test. He must pass an English exam to validate his diploma. With my foot, I'm used to it, I know how a CT scan goes, it should go pretty quickly. When the nurse returns after the exam is over, I can tell by her embarrassed smile and the intonation of her voice that something is wrong. I laughed nervously as I joined mum in the waiting room. No time to explain everything to him, the radiologist arrives.

- There are several anomalies. It's not nothing ... I took the initiative, you have an appointment Monday with a pulmonologist in the other hospital of Tours.

That is only three days later. Nothing reassuring, but I remain calm. There is no point in worrying until we know.

Everyone thinks about this long weekend. I'm going to the date determined to find out what I've got! With all of this unspoken, I have my list of possibilities with me.

I was far from suspecting that my parents and Flavien already had a clear idea of the diagnosis. Flavien, whose birthday is 30th of April, does not wish to be present and waits in the car. I am going to the meeting with my parents who have joined me. The doctor calmly asks us what we have understood and does not leave us in doubt for long.

- We're going to talk frankly… it's cancer.

A needle in a haystack

Often people say the sky fell on their heads when they heard it or the ground gave way beneath their feet. I didn't, as if I didn't realize or was ready to hear it when it wasn't a possibility I had noticed. I find myself saying only:

- This is crazy.

My parents are crying next to me.

- Will there be preservation of fertility? Asks my mother.
- You see far away mum.
- Precisely, this will be the first step to put in place. Retorts the pulmonologist.

An eleven-centimeter mass lodged between my heart and my lung, along with two small nodules next to it. She explains to me that whatever type of cancer you have to go through chemotherapy. Mum asks for my hospitalization, because I am very weak. As it is the day before bank holiday, the pulmonologist offers to digest the announcement with the family and come back in two days to hospitalize me and do a biopsy in my lung. We see Flavien waiting in the lobby of the hospital, he immediately understands, to our vexed heads, that his doubts are confirmed. I'm not crying, it hurts to make my parents, my boyfriend and ...

- Grandparents ! How will they react? I'm afraid something will happen to them with the shock of the news.

Straightforwardly, I announced it by message to my cousins and a few friends. At the time, I absolutely did not ask myself the question of whether or not this is the way to announce cancer.

> ### Hard prick
>
> "Oh no ! This is terrible!
> I hope you will get through this."

In two years, my body has developed two masses! One in my heel and now in the lung and each time on the left side. I keep telling myself, «This is crazy!». As soon as I feel another pain, I'm going to be scared ... It's a blow to everything! Especially since it's not my type to worry about my health, I am far from being a hypochondriac.

Flavien does not respond to calls from his relatives who want to wish him his birthday. They're bound to ask him how he's doing and he doesn't feel ready to explain the situation. We do not risk forgetting this date, it unfortunately falls badly ...

On Wednesday 2nd May, at 4 p.m. I was hospitalized in pulmonology. I arrive in a department on strike. On strike, but present. I am lucky to be in one of the few single rooms.

The next day, the pulmonologist and her team take a fiberoptic sample to determine the cancer. Lungs, thymus or lymphoma? I should have an early response at the end of the day. My throat is lightly anesthetized so that a long flexible tube passes through my mouth. I must not move despite my retching. They position the tube, it is an unusual and unpleasant sensation that a foreign body is moving towards his lung. Once positioned in the best position, with a «pistol» the needle grabs a fragment of flesh which they pull up by turning a crank to retrieve what they «fished». Seven samples are taken. But the pulmonologist asks me:

- We have access to another place, maybe only one of these samples can be examined. Do you agree to an eighth direct debit?

Now that I'm here ... I don't want to relive that painful moment again so since I can't speak, I lift my thumb in the air to agree. And I continue to crush the hand of the nurse standing next to me. When it's over, they tell me I was brave. I'm proud of myself, but I will never take such an exam again! Fortunately I hadn't inquired about the process otherwise I would have run away. When I come back to my room, I have no voice, as if I have screamed too much and I purr when I breathe. This makes me laugh. I take everything that happens to me as a new experience. I told myself I had nothing planned for the next few months anyway! Alone in my room, I reflect. It would be so incomprehensible if it was lung cancer. I have never smoked, I drink occasionally and very little. I'm not the party type and I don't abuse anything. I would almost define myself more as a granny who enjoys knitting in front of the television and gossiping with girlfriends. When I was 17 there was the cervical cancer vaccine awareness campaign. As this vaccine was recent, I remember very well telling my mother that she did not want to do it, because ...

- If I don't have this cancer, it will be another.

The same evening, under the pressure of the pulmonologist, the laboratory gave the first results. Normally, you have to wait at least one week. The pulmonologist comes to my room, sits next to me on the bed, and gently teaches me that two samples have been analyzed and that it is lymphoma.

- So it's not a cancer?
- It is, but it's better than lung cancer. It's definitely Hodgkin's lymphoma, but we have to wait for the biopsy details.

I don't know what lymphoma is. This is the first time I've heard this word. The next day, I change departments to go for onco-hemato. With two holidays and a weekend where nothing happens, my week in hospital is long. The service psychologist and art therapist are not present. In this department, the medical team is much more attentive, they take the time to talk, to reassure, to answer my questions. This service is well suited to long hospitalizations, the television is free, I can have various drinks and cookies. I also choose my meals. I find it hard to feel legitimate and accept these privileges. I don't feel sick and my first tears are oddly due to the fact that I do not pay for television and then, a few hours later, when I learn that I will no longer be able to donate my organs, I crack. I have had the donor card since I was 16. It was important to me to be useful when I died ... In a long time, a very long time!

After this interminable weekend, I meet my hematologist. Funny, it's named after the town where I was to take Flavien on a surprise weekend for his birthday. I refrain from telling him, because the moment is serious. She confirms that it is Hodgkin's lymphoma and asks me to name anything that could be a symptom of the disease.

- For many months now, when I only drink two sips of alcohol, I have had a really stiff stiffness in my left shoulder.

She explains to me that this is a typical Hodgkin sign, but that it's not common to feel it. My attending physician told me that it was most likely due to my fragile liver. Regarding my itchy patches on my face, this is also a symptom. In contrast, I never had any noticeable neck mass or weight loss or night sweats, just a little warmer at night.

How did I manage not to guess earlier? Whenever you look for two symptoms on the internet, you immediately come across the diagnosis of Hodgkin lymphoma. At the same time ... when you type anything that's going on in the body, you get diagnosed with cancer! And I'm not the type to panic before I have something concrete. As I find out, here's what I can read on the France Lymphome Espoir site: Hodgkin's lymphoma is cancer of the lymphatic network, the main component of the body's immune system. Hodgkin's disease accounts for 10% of all lymphomas and 1% of all cancers. It occurs in about 2,400 people per year. It most often affects young adults between the ages of 20 and 30. Hodgkin's disease is one of the most curable cancers, with over 80% cure being achieved. The exact causes of this disease are not known.

On 11th May, still hospitalized, I have an appointment for the preservation of fertility. In the waiting room, I am with two couples in their thirties. My large file in my arms, I shed a few tears, I don't really realize what I'm doing here. In the consultation room, I face a doctor and his intern. In an extremely serious tone, they explain the three possibilities to me:

- Surgical removal of an entire ovary for the freezing of fragments. This technique remains experimental to this day with less than a hundred pregnancies in the world. Or stimulation then sampling by puncture of the oocytes in local anesthesia. Or, I read in your file that you are in a relationship, you can do the follicular puncture with fertilization in order to freeze embryos.

I burst out laughing.

- Yeah, I can see myself saying this evening to my boyfriend «Hey, do you think that for our eleven months together we are freezing embryos?»

They remain stoic.

Do they realize they are talking to a 24 years old? Okay, some are ready or having children. But they don't ask me if that was in my plans. This meeting is disconcerting. I was hoping for a minimum of compassion or they laughed at my questionable humor. I come away stunned by this timeless exchange. I was not ready for this meeting, I should have gone with someone. This interview is the last, I am going home after ten days of hospitalization.

Very present on social networks I decided to announce it, because it will be part of my daily life for the next six months minimum and I do not intend to hide such a change in my life. I research Instagram in the hopes of finding someone with a similar story. For this I use #lymphome, #hodgkin, #lymphomedehodgkin. Many Germans post on #hodgkin. A whole community is open to me, it even has a name: the Kfighteuses. The K is the abbreviation for cancer in the medical field and fighteuse is fighter when it's frenchify. A majority of women have breast cancer. I find some great testimonials and decide to follow several.

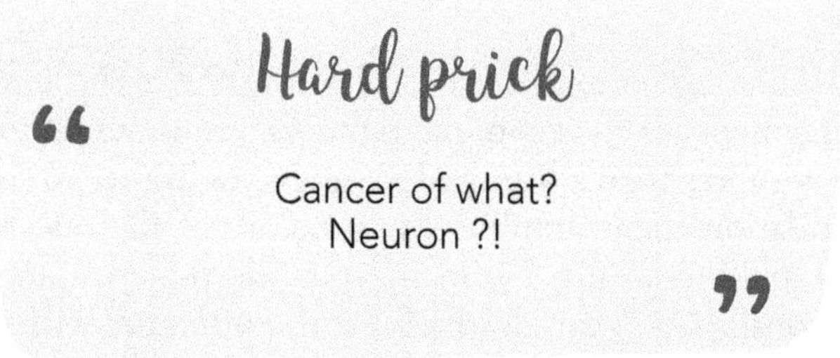

Wednesday 16th May, my cell phone rings, I have an appointment the next day at 7 am for the installation of the port-to-cath or also called an implantable chamber. It's a small box placed under the skin above my right breast that connects to the large vein in my heart. This allows chemo to be injected and preserves the veins in the arms. The PAC will also be used to take blood tests when I am hospitalized or to receive blood and platelets. I'm caught off guard, I wasn't expecting it so much that I'm on my way to spend a few days with my parents. I'm going anyway and dad will come with me to the hospital tomorrow.

There are about ten of us waiting on an outpatient basis, but only two for the installation of the PAC. A man speaks loudly and grumbles to his wife. After putting on a blouse, I go to a box where dad can wait with me. Around 9 a.m., the man exits the operating room, still moaning, it is finally my turn. I'm scared, I ask if someone can talk to me during the operation.

- I finish filling out the file on the computer and I arrive, reassures me the nurse.

But no one is coming! They give me an anesthetic injection in the chest and a few seconds after a serrated roller opens my skin ...

- I feel everything! Wait for the anesthesia to take effect!

The procedure continues after waiting a few microseconds. The surgeon pushes aside two sections of skin like a window. Without my glasses, I can't see anything around me, I start to cry, there is still no one around. This is a teaching hospital, the surgeon explains:

- So, don't let go of the tube, otherwise it goes into the artery of the heart.

- Well great! I answer to try to start a conversation. But the doctor ignores me and continues to explain internally.

No, but go ahead, pretend I'm not present, I'm grieving inside. When it's time to sew up, the nurse finally comes to me and finds me in tears, she doesn't understand. It's so painful, I'm angry. Dad joins me, I want to cry in anger, but it hurts too much for that. Zero humanity! They do this manipulation every day, but for me it was a big step! And dreaded!

Few people talk about the cruelty of fitting the PAC, because everything quickly follows, tomorrow is the much anticipated PET Scan. A scanner that can locate the various inflammations in 3D and assess the extent of the disease. It's a test that lasts three to four hours, is painless and requires an empty stomach.

I let myself be guided serenely. I leave my things in the locker room and keep the key with me, I have the right to take my phone. I'm waiting on a stretcher in a room, alone. The nurse infuses my arm as the contrast medium may clog the PAC. I wait half an hour before the doctor comes to ask me a few questions and explain the procedure to me. Then the nurse returns and stands behind a glass cart to inject me with the radioactive product contained in a three kilogram lead «capsule». I stay alone while the product diffuses into my body. The time is long and I am starting to feel hungry. Next time I'll pick up a book. After fifty minutes, the caregiver comes to pick me up to go to the bathroom before the exam. She then directs me to a small room where I have to remove anything metallic on me. Skinny, my pants and top have a zipper so I put on a skinny blouse. I also take off my glasses and someone picks me up. Again, without glasses I can't see anything, I can see a smile, but it's quite disturbing. I lie down and the person covers me with a sheet to keep me from getting cold. After 15-20 minutes, in the scanner, a new person helps me stand up and hands me a blue card. As I get dressed, I read that you should drink plenty of water to urinate as often as possible and avoid close and prolonged contact with young children or pregnant women for twelve hours. I have a snack before leaving; a glass of grenadine and a strawberry-filled madeleine. Now that this exam is done, I can have cortisone to alleviate the effects, such as my headaches and my facial plaques.

The same evening, my daily punctures begin in the lower part of my stomach, to develop several follicles for the purpose of retrieving my oocytes. My home nurse has to come between 6 and 8 p.m. for ten days. During the entire treatment, it is advisable to avoid endocrine disruptors: washing products, insecticides ... I inquire about the pain of the sample by local anesthesia in a Facebook group that talks about IVF routes. Most young women choose general anesthesia. My two previous painful examinations and the rest of the treatment course being uncertain, I do not want to repeat the experience and I ask for a general anesthesia. The doctor grants it to me without my having to negotiate. I know that performing local anesthesia saves them time, but my physical and psychological pain is important at the moment. If my only goal had been to have a child, I would certainly have agreed to take this sample using local anesthesia because it was less invasive and faster. But my mission is elsewhere.

Every other day, I have a check-up in the hospital; a blood test, then an ultrasound by endovaginal probe. On the first day, we are the first with Flavien, from 7:30 am! They told us to plan three hours on site and indeed we go out at past ten.

To get to the hospital, we pass the high school where I did my diploma Graphic Industries. I loved my studies in printing, I look back on it with a lot of nostalgia, because it was the time of discovering independence, freedom and recklessness.

I am very upset, I sleep poorly, everything bothers me. I want to throw everything out the window and me! Maybe it's the hormones. To calm myself down, I listen to *Hoshi* and his current track *Ta Marinière*. During the check-up on 28th May, I have four large oocytes on each side and small ones that still need to grow. The stimulation is enough to trigger ovulation tomorrow. This is another injection to be given at set times, for me at 9:10 pm Ovulation occurs 37 to 40 hours after this injection, which is why the puncture is done 36 hours after the injection. On the night of 30-31th May, I had such severe stomach cramps that I almost passed out. In the morning, I am better and Flavien drops me off very early at the hospital to have my oocyte retrieval. The procedure is quick, it lasts ten minutes. I wake up painlessly and glad I asked for general anesthesia. When the surgeon tells me that they have collected eight oocytes of which «only» seven are viable for freezing, I wonder.

- That makes a child and a half?
- Whether you want a child or not, a single good chance is better than zero. Your eggs will be 24 years old forever.

It should be taken into account that during «thawing» some oocytes will be lost. Then about half of the oocytes will give embryos. I am an only child and I regret it, I would have liked to have siblings. Until now, I have always said that if I had children it would be two or none. But his speech gives me an electric shock that changes my way of seeing things. Maybe in the end I don't want a child? It's good to have the opportunity to change your mind. My attending physician also appeases all my questions. She advises me not to do a fertility test after the treatments are finished.

- Life is amazing and a test can put some misconceptions in our head.

I totally agree with his reasoning.

Now that my oocytes are freeze, I start a pill that aims to put me in menopause and preserve my ovaries. It is a progestin that blocks ovulation. This will prevent my bleeding and the red blood cells from falling.

Before my first chemo, the hospital advises me to shorten my hair that reaches the middle of my back, to be less hassle when it comes time to fall.

- Great, this is your chance to donate hair again!

Indeed, in May 2017 I made a donation to the Solid'Hair association, which collects the hair and sells it to wigmakers. The money raised is redistributed to cancer patients to help fund a wig. A quality wig is expensive, on average 500 euros for a short cut and social security only reimburses 125 euros.

Fate wanted it to be a year later that I was told of my cancer. So I go back to Nathalie's hair salon with whom I made my first hair donation. It's an even more emotional moment than the first time, but she knows how to comfort me with her kindness. I can donate because I am donating twenty-five centimeters in length and my hair is not colored. There is another french association, *Fake hair don't care*, which collects strands from ten centimeters even when they are dyed.

But I can hardly accept this new haircut, I who have always had long hair, now that I am four inches on my head, I do not recognize myself. I'm sad. I really didn't think I would react like that. I reason with myself, it's okay, it's just hair. When I'm bald, I already know I don't want a wig. It wouldn't be me, I'd be scared of feeling disguised and I didn't want her scratching me and being uncomfortable. Still, being bald is a strong marker of illness, but I don't intend to shamefully hide it, I haven't done anything wrong. I will rather go on turbans. The hospital gave me a brochure, but the models are dated. Fortunately, on the internet, I spotted two nice and flowery ones that I will be receiving in a few days.

Sewing needle

Only a few days before my first chemo, the weather is fine, we see friends, family, we have dinner in a good restaurant to celebrate our first year together with Flavien. I have been told that I will definitely lose my appetite and being a very greedy foodie I am making the most of it.

From the booklet the nurse gave me explaining Hodgkin's lymphoma, I deduce from reading that I am in stage 3 or 4. There are four stages in Hodgkin's disease, the first being weaker. At the hospital, I asked not to know him ... anyway, it's a cancer that can be treated well, especially in young people. Despite everything, this information runs through my head.

The day before my first chemo, I need to take care of my mind! Flavien helps me sew until late. I'm very afraid that everything will stop tomorrow, that I will no longer be able to do anything. I love creative hobbies and I really pity my knitting, my sewing machine and all my needles.

At 24 years old do you really know what chemotherapy is? I only remember the image of my neighbor's mother when we were little, weakened, pale complexion, a felt hat on her head. That was almost twenty years ago, treatments have evolved, they are said to be less aggressive.

Last week, I met the hospital's announcement nurse. She explained to me the possible side effects and the different products I would be receiving. Chemotherapy is not a drug, but a set of drugs called treatment, there are as many of them as cancers. My protocol is called BEACOPP. Five products will be injected between fifteen minutes and two hours with the addition of a pill of chemo and cortisone. I must have six cycles, each cycle is twenty-one days. I will be hospitalized for three days then one day the following week. This promises an explosive cocktail! I can have nausea and vomiting, but several medications are planned to remedy it. I can get mucositis and canker sores so I have baking soda mouthwashes to do. I need to avoid exposure to the sun and protect my skin when I go out.

D-Day ! Wednesday 6th June 2018.

My special chemo bag has been ready for days. For the occasion, I'm wearing my pretty beige dress with black polka dots, the one that gives me confidence and that I could wear every day for the past few weeks because I feel so good in it. I arrive at the hospital at 10 am, with Flavien. The reception directs us to the first floor in the weekday service, which I discover. Room 15, at the end of the hall, is bright even though I have a view of a building under construction.

The nurse sticks a numbing patch on «my little box» so I won't feel anything after an hour when placing the catheter needle. I'm not afraid of needles, but this is unusual as a system. Alone with the nurse, we have to wear a mask. She sets up a «sterile drape» on a table, she unfolds a paper «tablecloth», she puts many hoses, compresses, products on it ... She puts on gloves, disinfects my skin where the PAC is located and asks me to inhale and then block my breath.

- I'm stinging! Are you okay?
- Oh ! I hardly felt a thing, it's fast!

She does a vein return, to see if the blood is coming through the PAC and to make sure that the product is going to flow properly. Everything's fine, she can hook up the plastic hoses, one of which is connected to a hydration bag. The PAC must be constantly «powered» at the risk of it becoming clogged. The hose that goes from my PAC and that I have to keep "plugged in" for the three days is connected to an infusion stand. From there start several pipes for the different infusions or the different bags. Yes, it is complex! Fortunately, this foot is on wheels, so it can follow me everywhere.

Mum joins us at the start of the afternoon, I haven't had my chemo yet, the three of us are waiting. The intern comes to ask me many questions for my file. I also wrote down questions in my little notebook. I do not hesitate to express all my questions. I ask her permission to use essential oils without swallowing them, as I have read that this may help me to alleviate several side effects. He gives me the authorization after consulting the pharmacists at the hospital. Glad I can use essential oils, it's more natural than medicine, it's good that they're open to it in this hospital.

It's 4 pm, the afternoon shift is coming in and with them the first bag of chemo. I recognize the caregiver! He is a friend of my friend's best friend. I call out to him, it calms me to «know» someone, because I was a little lost. The nurse returns, without the slightest sign of empathy, and sets up a machine on the «drip stand». It's a box of about twenty centimeters, a pump to be exact. It blocks the hose from the chemo bag there, the machine will adjust the flow and signal with a sound if there is an air bubble and when everything is drained. I turn to mum and Flavien and tell them I want to cry. Nicole, a friend of mum's, who offers good advice, suggested that I imagine the product as light diffusing through my body attacking bad cells and then expelling them. The first product is orange, it's surprising. While the bag slowly empties, Élodie, the art therapist, introduces herself. Her visit takes my mind off things, she wears a colorful outfit and smiles broadly. Its goal is to bring art in general into the lives of patients. Art therapy is part of the supportive care offered to patients. She reassures me that I can continue with manual activities and she will help me with this when I am hospitalized. I also meet Ismérie, the social worker, who answers my financial questions. I should only lose a third of my salary. It's not a concern of mine, I know it will and that my parents can help me if I need to. I am lucky to be in France to be treated and not to pay for my treatments or hospitalizations.

Flavien came back to the apartment and at 5:30 p.m. he sends me a message:

- Weird I was hungry ... Normal I did not eat this afternoon.

Poor guy, with the stress, waiting for chemo, he didn't even go to the hospital cafeteria to eat anything.

I discover the shrill noise made by the machine… the first product is finished, I'm fine. A product follows to protect my bladder, the nurse warns me that I will be urinating a lot. An hour later comes the second chemo, it makes me feel like my head and jaw are in a vise. Looks like serious things are starting. The last pocket is placed at 9 p.m. Mum helps me put on my pajamas and walks away. I feel like I'm knocked out, trying to fall asleep, but it's like the disease is telling me, «No, stay awake!» I have a hot sweat then a cold one and my stomach hurts. My perspiration is heavy and it smells like medicine. I try to come to terms with it and tell myself that my body is defending itself from everything it received today. I can't concentrate on anything, I'm just in terrible pain.

At 1:01 am, I send a message to mum «Hi, it's not going well». I don't know what to wear anymore and I decide to call the nurses, it's the night shift. They don't try to understand, barely speak to me and give me a pain reliever, *Acupan*. But I have to face the facts, the pain is stronger than the pain killer. I fall asleep around 5 a.m. and wake up at 7 a.m. by the construction of the building next door.

Breakfast is served at 8:30 am I'm angry after the work. The nurse puts a waterproof bandage on my PAC and asks me if I am fit enough to go to the shower on my own.

- Yes, I will only wash my body, because I have read about not washing your hair four to eight days after chemo.
- Ahah! You must have read this on the internet!

I grab my green binder given by the announcement nurse and find the phrase that gives this advice. The ! I nailed his beak!

One of my best friends, Noémie, agreed to visit me in the hospital. I wasn't sure how this second day of chemo was going to go so she was kind enough to come. When she arrived I felt her pissed off, she's a speedy person, but usually always interested in others and this time she was furnishing the conversation by mostly talking about herself. I don't think she saw that the chemo was leaking, that the orderly came to clean the room, and that my dark circles spoke volumes about my previous night.

My chemo for the day lasts two hours. Even though I haven't slept much, my nerves are holding me back. I am so hydrated that I will pee every 30 minutes.

Daddy's coming to pick me up on Friday. We leave the hospital at 3:30 p.m. after the last drug identical to yesterday. I come home tired, but not too sick. I point out to dad that my hair texture is strange. I haven't washed them since Wednesday morning, but they don't have the texture of dirty or greasy hair, they seem… elastic. I have an overwhelming amount of medicine to take per day, including pill chemo for a week. We collected a whole box of drugs from the pharmacy! Especially fifteen boxes of *Paracetamol* ...

- I'll be able to sell some! I say jokingly.

It's hot in the apartment! I'm completely exhausted, but I accept that one of my best friends will drop by quickly.

- You're all dapper! he takes me out when he arrives.

It's awkward, but I apologize, he is certainly confused by the situation because he tries more jokes than usual.

This morning, Monday 11th June, I am exhausted and as if disconnected from my body. After a little nap, things get better, I want to take the opportunity to go buy a book on cancer at the library. I arrive in a shelf, at random, books are put forward on the table including a block entitled CANCER in big, bold and red. Perfect ! I take this one. The caption reads «What if our emotions could heal us?» »Doctor Julien Drouin's book speaks to me. For me cancer is caused by emotions, I missed my body's warning messages and now I have cancer. But why and how? I can tell my body hurts when I'm sad or angry. I would like to understand what is going on, how and why my body has developed these masses.

This Wednesday is day 8 of the cycle, I'm on the same weekday shift for the day. I arrive at 10 a.m. and the medical team offers to meet the socio-esthetician. She gives me a hand massage and then a manicure. But I see the clock ticking and maybe my chemo has arrived so I'm not enjoying the moment. It's a shame, because it's only after a meal, at 1 pm, that I receive my product. It will initiate the aplasia phase, which is the destruction of white blood cells. My head is spinning and I have painful stomach cramps, but I'm glad to come home to rest. The days go by and I don't feel any physical effects from this drop in white blood cells. I am even quite in good shape. I get subcutaneous injections of growth factors, to stimulate the bone marrow. The only way to check the growth of white blood cells is to have your blood drawn, so I have two a week. After five days of belly pricks, I start to feel pain in the muscles or maybe the bones, from my hips to my calves. As well as a big headache and a sore jaw. Canker sores appear, despite mouthwashes with baking soda. As all of these symptoms scare me, I call the ward and the doctor offers to come to the hospital. I live 15 minutes from the hospital, which is very convenient. A nurse connects me to the PAC to take a blood test and be hydrated while waiting for the results. A few hours later ... More fear than harm, it's my white blood cells that suddenly increased and causing this pain. I have nothing else to do but wait. Except patience isn't really my thing. I am curious, I like to discover, to be constantly in action. What a frustration not to be able to do anything! I try to read a few lines, but my eyes quickly blur.

It's been two weeks since I had my first chemo and I'm starting to lose my hair. They get stuck on my brush and it's worse when I run my hand through my hair. It does have a funny effect though… I could believe myself in a scene from a movie, it is so unreal. I wait three more days before calling Nathalie, my hairdresser. I really wanted to be ready to shave them and this time I am. I find it everywhere, I'm sick of it. I go outside, and run my hand through my hair a lot of times, I see it flying all around me. We have so much on our heads that it could last a long time. I have fun cutting my bangs. This is a bad idea since I have a cob. At least I will have tried and that makes me laugh. Nathalie kindly offered to come and shave my hair at home after work. It's an emotional moment, especially for Flavien, who wanted to be there. But my smile instantly returns when I look at myself, in the mirror, without hair. I like ! I don't scare myself!

Dad doesn't want to see me bald. I'm a little upset because Flavien and Mum accept it and don't find it shocking and I love myself that way too. I explain to him that he will not be able to «escape» it: it is hot and if I sleep at their place, he will see me in the morning. After a few days of reflection, he accepts. I was born with a full hair, so we will have discovered my bald head at least once.

Besides my hair, I had to part with my ring and my perfume. The first squeezes my finger too much and I can't stand the second, it gives me headaches.

21th of June, it's Music Day… Bah! I don't really want to sing! I received my first report. I read it on my own and learn that I am in stage IV b, the highest. Even though I had a little idea, I had asked not to know him. Okay ... let's say I couldn't escape it, eventually I would have known.

Wednesday 27th June, start of the second cycle. 4 pm, room 12, I breathe my peppermint essential oil to avoid nausea. The caregiver takes my temperature, my blood pressure ... all the usual checks when entering the room. A second caregiver takes inventory of my personal belongings, although I don't plan to set foot outside this room during the three days. She also makes me choose my meals. I have the choice between four starters, four main courses, two dairy products and one piece of fruit or one yogurt. Last time around, I selected balanced meals, but this time, in order to be able to swallow everything, I decide to only eat foods that make me happy. That is to say mainly starchy foods.

The treatment bags are being prepared in the hospital, while waiting for the first chemo product to arrive, I ask the art therapist. A filthy drawing that I have just tried makes me cry. I feel bad. My reaction unsettles me and I realize that I am crying about something else. I tell him that I read the stage of the cancer on the report sheet. Twenty minutes later, the information was transmitted and I am surprised to see the manager arrive in my room. He reassures me and explains to me that I should not be alarmed, that they need this number to communicate quickly between doctors.

It's already time for the second pocket. The one where I lose my footing. Going to the bathroom every 30 minutes, I watch my face change, it's dull and tired, my eye area is dark and sunken, a real panda face, and my neck is swelling. I seem lucid, but the next day I don't remember the discussions. Luckily, have my mum stay with me until 9 p.m., she'll help me put on my pajamas and can tell me what happened. In oncology, there are no visiting hours unlike other departments where it is only from 2 p.m. to 6 p.m. This allows me to organize a visit from my loved ones when I am the least tired and when I need it.

Another complicated first night, this time it's confirmed it's not stress. I feel sick again, three hours after the end of the product, and I fall asleep at 4 in the morning. This does not prevent the night nurse, absolutely not listening to me, from saying:

- This is anxiety! I can only offer you a *Xanax*.

Even for a headache I rarely take medication, but in desperation I accept Xanax, you never know. Obviously, that doesn't change anything. I take my pain patiently. My pain, patience ... the expression takes on its full meaning. I suspect that there is nothing you can do for ailment caused by a chemical product. I would have liked listening and compassion from him. Let her reassure me by telling me that it is normal with the large dose of the product that I am injected on the first day.

On Thursdays, the only thing that tempts me is the praline cream like the one I ate last night. The caregiver does several services to find me. She comes back to my room proud of her, pot in hand, I am touched by this little attention!

- I have a second one that I'm putting in the fridge with your name on it. Do not hesitate !

I hear the afternoon shift starting to arrive. Not missed! The caregiver I know arrives to continue the conversation from last night, but ... I have no recollection of it! It's his last week and I have asked him to have some chocolates to bring to his colleagues tomorrow. So, even in the doldrums, I ask for something to eat ...

Flavien is checking the medication prescription the intern gave me. He compares with that of the first cycle and realizes that it misses the *Natulan*. The chemo in cachet! The *Solupred* is also missing! A derivative of cortisone. Basically, the intern forgot a lot! What if this had been my first chemo? Would I have left the hospital without my chemo pills? I am angry and the good thing about anger is that it keeps me in good shape. I let everyone who comes into my room know that I'm pissed off at the resident who gave the prescription. But why didn't she compare with the first prescription?

Otherwise, the injection of the only product of the day goes well.

The student caregiver knocks on my door to… give me a nice bowl with good chocolates! I wasn't asking for so much, I was very touched by the attention. He wishes me the best for the future.

It's the same soup tonight as yesterday, but it's not going through.

The cortisone works, instead of sleeping I write a list of the hundred things I want to accomplish in my notebook. Eat pizza in Italy and fries in Belgium, ride a horse on the beach, go to Alsace at Christmas, have an orchard, adopt a cat ...

Friday 29th June, I have red patches that itch and heat. After the doctor's visit, the nurse injects me with an antiallergenic which knocks me out. I'm frozen over 30 degrees!

First week of July, a week where I felt sad and upset. I didn't think I could feel any worse. It is exhaustion that hurts the body and medication or naps do not change it. It is unlike any other fatigue, it is truly unique, it's hard to describe it to my loved ones. It's not the same as after a day's work or the night after. I'm exhausted, my body weighs a ton.

Thursday 5th July, the analysis laboratory calls me at 8:30 pm to advise me to go to the emergency room, because my neutrophils, a category of white blood cells, are at 120 instead of 1,700. haemato told me to avoid any risk of infection, so going to the emergency room would be like going into the mouth of the wolf.

I contact my oncologist who is still in the hospital, she explains to me that I am in what is called aplasia. I have to limit contact, not go to a mall and be very careful about what I eat, like a pregnant woman would. For example, it is advisable to drink bottled water to avoid bacteria. I am not allowed to make homemade rillettes, or unpasteurized cheeses. It's a shame when you know the reputation of the rillettes from Tours and the goat cheese from Sainte-Maure-de-Touraine. Lots of restrictions like these are going to push me to the end of my patience. To put it simply, we have stocked of frozen food, it helps prevent germs as much as possible. I discover with pleasure their dishes. It must be said that I have no problem eating, quite the opposite, I have a *stomach on legs* and I am delighted when someone invites me to eat. Food is my grandparents' big concern!

- Do you at least eat? they question me constantly.

The psychologist explains to me that this is the first worry a parent has when it comes to motherhood. The baby can only come out if he has gained a good weight. A good appetite is a sign of good health. Doctors make sure you keep your weight off and with the cortisone and liters of fluid injected I even tend to swell.

The next morning, I'm on the floor, hanging on the toilet bowl to vomit. Flavien is about to leave to take his TOEIC, but he doesn't want to go any more so as not to leave me alone, given my condition.

- There is nothing to do, it will pass. Take your exam, it's important!

My vomits brought him luck, because he came home very happy, he thinks he has passed his TOEIC. At the end of the day, the call from the training center confirmed this. A good thing done ! Bravo Flavien!

Two days later my gum hurts, *Paracetamol* doesn't do anything so I put peppermint essential oil on my skin, it cools and relieves me.

10th July, go I'm better, I must take advantage before starting the third cycle. I see some friends, with Flavien we go out when it's not too hot, I rest my heavy body in the hammock and above all we celebrate Flavien's diploma with his family and my parents. These are good times and I feel like I live them more intensely than if I wasn't sick. I'm really enjoying it because I know the respite is short-lived.

For my second PET Scan, Monday 16th July at 2 p.m., I'm not fooled, I'm equipped: pants without zippers and a top without anything metallic. I also took a book with me. The nurse tries to prick my arm twice before handing over. But it's not a success with that other nurse trying to prick the hand. So they get together, they pat my hand, make me clench my fist harder, move the tourniquet, I run my arm under the hot water… I make jokes with a broad smile to relax me, but the tests s ‘continue and I start to tremble, tears come to my eyes. The seventh time is the right one! Relief. Seven attempts to infuse me! Seven times! I've always had thin veins and the first two chemos did not help. At 5 p.m., I leave the exam. Flavien is on the phone in the waiting room. In view of the hour and my craving for savory, we headed to a great bakery that serves good sweet and savory things all day. Comfortably seated in a large leather armchair, the perfect place to relax. It's nice ...

We don't tell ourselves enough that we are lucky when our bodies are doing well. But I'm worried about future pain, so Flavien keeps telling me:

- Day after day.

Prick of boost

I start the third cycle of treatment with my red blood cells at 8. This is low since the norm is between 11 and 14 g / dL. So I am very weak. The nurse wonders why a transfusion is not scheduled before the chemo. But with my fatigue, the discussion ends there. Despite my lethargic state, as soon as a caregiver walks into my room and asks me, «Are you okay? »I always answer« Yes ». I am taken back by mum who qualifies my remarks. I like interacting with the teams so much that I don't want to waste time and prefer to talk about light topics. Anyway, for a few months now, the «Are you okay?» «No longer makes sense to me. Sometimes I don't even respond. It is an automatism, used by all, to be polite. Who really cares about the answer? Moreover, this question leaves little choice: yes or no. Ditto for «Hope you are well» it annoys me and I want to say «keep hoping». I prefer to be asked «How are you?» That gives information, because it is neither all white nor all black. I'm quibbling, but with cancer I find the subject important, so my answer is:

- I'm tired, but I'm in good spirits!

No doubt, it's the summer vacation, few caregivers are present in the department. Besides, there is no doctor on duty, it is the mess. I asked the intern for the PET scan results, which he brought to me a few minutes later without explanation. We can decipher that I have moved to stage II and the disease is on the decline. This is good news, we are relieved. The usual treatments follow one another ... I feel like throwing up, I'm hot and cold, my over-iced iced tea is helping me a lot.

The first night is still complicated for my body, I fall asleep around 4 a.m. The next day, it is still very calm in the ward, the psychologist will come to see me, but above all I will be able to rest.

Friday morning, I ask for a blood test to check my hemoglobin. I prefer to have my blood drawn in the hospital, as the nurse takes it directly from my PAC so I don't feel a thing. The doctor tells me it's useless, it won't have changed in three days, but she accepts. My chemo ends at 3 p.m. so I can go home, but first I think about claiming the results of my blood test. A few minutes later, an energetic young woman comes into my room and announces:

- We'll put two bags of blood on you!

Already gone in the opposite direction, she adds that she will tell my doctor.

- Who was it ? Am I going to be transfused? Has it gone down? I didn't follow it all there!

After more than an hour of waiting, no explanation ... I'm still plugged in and decide to go to the ward next door myself, where my hematologist's office is. She informs me that the intern who went to my room did not warn her and that in addition to that she went home ... I'm at 7.7, it has indeed dropped, she approves the transfusion, but a bag of blood. This is going to be my first blood transfusion. I take it as an additional experience in my adventure.

The transfusion lasts 1 hour 30 minutes, the nurse is watching me closely, especially my fever which could be a sign that I cannot stand the transfusion. I am not alone, Flavien is by my side and my parents have joined us. It feels weird to think that someone else's blood is adding to yours. It's even stranger when I want pineapple juice and the nurse's aide brings me grape juice that is exactly the same color as the blood bag. We all laugh about it together. But I don't forget my annoyance: it's crazy that we have to watch everything, claim everything. I wonder how old people do, alone and too tired to control everything.

Wednesday 25th July, day 8 in a day hospital, on the ground floor of the hospital, the place where everything goes faster, too fast, and where there are more of us. It's a hell of a lot less fun, everyone is in a rush and urgent, the caregivers don't have time to talk. And I love to talk! Fortunately, there is always Flavien, mum or dad to accompany me. I come in very weak, mum thinks they are not going to give me my chemo, but after checking my constants, the chemo is validated. However, it started badly, I forgot to put my anesthetic patch on my implantable chamber before leaving. This presents me with a big dilemma, either I ask one, but I have to wait an hour for it to take effect, or the nurse pricks my PAC without the skin being anesthetized. I am panicked, I start to cry. I want to stay in the hospital as short as possible, but I'm afraid of the pain.

- Sometimes you have to do it without a patch. The patients aren't that bad, the nurse reassures me.

I accept to save time and prove to myself that I am courageous. It is indeed more stressful than painful. But it's not a pleasant feeling so I will try not to forget my numbing patch again before I get to the hospital the next few times! But if it has to happen again, I won't panic.

Besides, courage ... A person who chooses to refuse treatment at the risk of his life is courageous. I am not courageous when I undergo my treatments, at the limit I would say that I have strength and hope, that is what makes me persevere! However, according to the dictionary, courage is «moral strength; acts in spite of difficulties». So okay maybe I have a little courage.

> «A strong person is not a person who never falls,
> a strong person is a person who falls and gets up.»

The chemo is on, I doze off, wrapped in my blanket despite the summer heat. The young intern from the day hospitalization department brings me a PET scan report.

- I already had this paper last week, I indicate.

She shrugs her shoulders and leaves. Mum is decoding the mail to wait. Surprised, she shouts at me:

- It's not the same report at all! Stage III!

I ring the orderly and ask to see a doctor. The doctor does not take long to arrive in the room… We want an explanation!

- The hemato intern printed out what was on the computer, which was a report that had not yet been proofread and signed by the imaging doctor. It's okay Ms. Naudin, your PET scan is still good, don't worry.

Shortly after, I had an appointment with my hematologist, I took the opportunity to ask him to see the PET scan images. She makes sure I'm ready and explains the scanner to me. I really see a lot of «black spots» on my left chest, less than two months ago, sure, but still!

The days go by and I have the pictures in my head. I think I just realize I'm sick. I've been less serene since then, but maybe it's a good thing to realize what's going on. I now know where the chemo works in my body.

Granocyte bites, to boost my white blood cells, hurt my bones too much. Pain like I was growing up and nothing could calm her down. Until now, the hospital had suggested that I take paracetamol, but I searched the internet and reading patient testimonials and asked my hematologist for *Zarzio* shots. If I hadn't inquired, the hospital would not offer me this alternative. For them it's the same product, however with these new bites I hardly have any pain! I had three blood tests the week after my eighth day of treatment to keep my white blood cell count well under control. It's a relief, it allows me to cope better with the period of aplasia.

I finally know how to tie my scarves nicely on my head. I'm glad I found a technique that was simple enough so as not to tire my arms too much.

Instant scarf knotting:

I put the unfolded scarf over my head with one-third of the fabric on one side on the shoulder and the remaining two-thirds on the other shoulder. I join the two pieces on the back of my head and cross them. The longest, I iron it over my bald head and finish by tying the two pieces of fabric together with a classic knot on the side of my head. I love !

Two mornings in a row when I vomit, I feel weak, but I do not feel great pain. My red blood cells are at 7.9 normally I should have a transfusion. But the hospital lets me know I'm young, I can wait. They gave me Ferritin tablets to increase the iron in my blood and I started the *EPO* shots which are supposed to stimulate the production of red blood cells. More bites! Although these are more painful, it's only once a week and I don't have bruises on my stomach yet. There is also the «natural» method which consists in eating more protein, it is found in large quantities in red meat ... But for this to be effective on the production of red blood cells, I would have to eat it bleeding, which is contraindicated during treatment since the risk of bacteria is high. This is not the only dietary inconsistency, grapefruit should be avoided during treatment because it causes interactions, and yet the hospital serves it. They also serve us white beans while the chemos cause digestive problems.

The home nurse comes between 11 am and 3 pm ... I can't wait to go to sleep. When she finally arrives, she finds me weak and worried, so she takes my pulse which is 113 beats per minute instead of 90. In the evening, the nurse comes home distraught. She saw the result and told me to contact my hematology department immediately. This time the red blood cells are extremely low: 6.9. I am so weak that even going to the bathroom is difficult. So I am not immune to the transfusion on 31st July. In addition to the two bags of blood, I'm allowed a 30-minute platelet bag and antibiotics to treat my cold that has been going on for weeks.

A hell of a boost that allows me to cook and watch the entire movie on television tonight, despite spending seven hours in the hospital. In summer, there are fewer blood donations, so the wait is longer to receive a compatible blood bag. The good thing about platelets is that they can be received from any donor, the blood type doesn't matter.

I stay locked up for several days because of the heat outside. Can't keep the apartment cool, it's over 30 degrees inside. Already when I don't like summer, I feel like I can't handle the heat so well since the treatments, it's difficult. I dream of going to the craft shop. Clothing stores are not really my thing. I have a strange obsession with the night markets, I ask Flavien to go to everyone in the area. In the evening, it is cooler. I have nothing else to think about, therefore I develop fads. The most obsessive is the food. Right now, I really feel like going crazy, I think about it all day and even at night. It's been forever since I ate this round bun topped with parsley butter, rillettes and more. A delicious local specialty! However, I have more and more difficulty with food in the hospital. The treatments amplify my sense of smell and everything there makes me nauseous, especially their white bread. I can't eat salad anymore, yet it is tasteless. I eat peaches and luckily the hospital has some in stock!

You don't get used to chemo, it gets harder and harder with each session. I'm so scared of the fourth cycle starting tomorrow! I've asked to see the hypnotherapist to help me get through the first night better, but she won't be available. So is the psychologist and art therapist who are on vacation.

To relax, we go to the cinema with Flavien. Despite the film being only 1h45, I realize that I have the concentration of a 4 year old. I'm sick of it, it's long, I can't wait to get out, I can't sit still, the sound is deafening. I WANT TO GO HOME.

8th August, room 18… When to go…

There is a good atmosphere in the corridors. When a patient leaves their room, even if they are bald, they are dressed in a big smile. They are usually old people, but I never see young people my age. The nurse explains to me that they do like me, they stay in their rooms. There is a hospital for children and then a hospital for adults, but nothing has been thought of for young adults. I would be interested in interacting with young people, outside of social media. Even if the latter are very useful.

At the end of the first day, the last product flows out slowly. I'm on the phone with grandma, my throat is starting to sting. I cut the conversation short and start to cough, my throat is swelling, I ring, I choke more and more, I look at mum with wide eyes of incomprehension.

Sarah, the caregiver, comes into my room and immediately understands. Within seconds, she takes Mum out of the bedroom to make way for the nurse who immediately stops the product and injects me with medicine to stop the swelling in my throat. I just had an allergic reaction to the second product. It had gone well the first few times! The same chemo is restarted one hour, under surveillance.

I always slept alone during my hospitalizations, but this time I asked mum to stay with me the first night. I can relax my body from the constant itching on my back. Hoshi's album is on repeat. I don't think she'll be able to hear it anymore. I have noticed that some music soothes the body and limits my pain. That's why I created an SOS playlist when I'm feeling sick inside.

SOS Vol. 1
Playlist
LECTURE ALÉATOIRE
Ta marinière
Hoshi
Comment je vais faire
Hoshi
Demain
Bigflo & Oli X Petit Biscuit
Pour oublier
Kendji Girac
La même
Maître Gims, Vianney

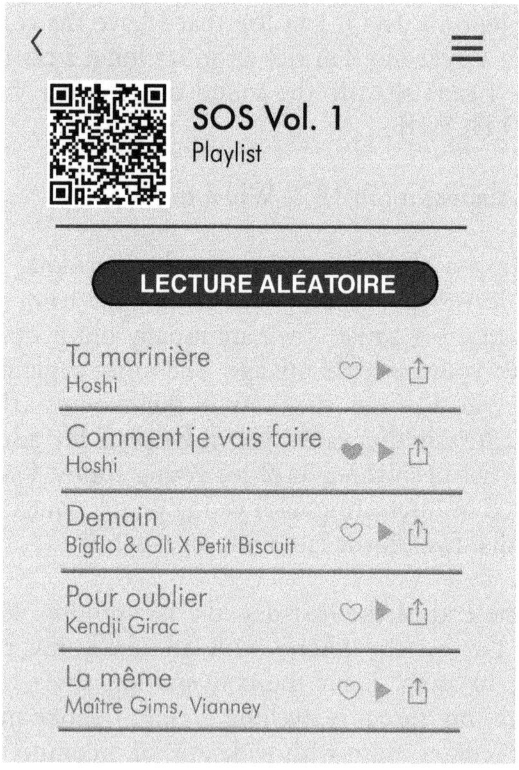

Mum dozes off a few times, but I wake her up by begging to keep the itching. It is only at 2:30 am that I fall asleep, which is nevertheless earlier than the previous cycles.

Apparently it's hot in my room, but I'm really cold from the chemo. The intern arrives and gives me two pieces of information:

- Day 8 of the cycle falls on 15th August, a bank holiday, so the treatment is postponed until the next day. And your next cycle will certainly be smoother if you switch to ABVD.

The change in protocol is classic for Hodgkin lymphoma. If after two or four BEACOPP chemo the results are good, the "milder" chemo is considered.

The second day ends, I am tired. I had a visit from Nicole. He was one of the few people who offered to come see me. But in the evening, when I'm alone in my room, I wonder about the impact of shifting day 8. I share my concern with the nurse who does his last turn before giving way to the night shift. .

- Yes, it is very serious, it will cause the healing to fail! You can go home tonight, that's no use anymore, but you're already healed anyway so it's okay!

I'm in a bad mood and I don't want to understand this humor... I just wanted it to reassure me.

6.30 am, the noise pollution generated by construction work serves as my alarm clock. Two hours later, while I am still drowsy, the nurse rinses my PAC to «unclog the plumbing.» It gives me a salty taste in my mouth, not pleasant before breakfast. In addition, the nurse plans to start my chemo at 9 a.m. Except that the chemo products affect the taste, I want to have my breakfast quietly before the third day of treatment starts and I can't eat anything at noon. In addition, it is recommended to wait 24 hours between the two chemos. Corn…

- You are young, you put up with it well, we can go more than 2 hours from yesterday, try to convince me the nurse to save time on her schedule.

After strong protests from me, she puts down chemo at 10:30 am I tend to share what I think and feel, sometimes without thinking. This is more the case with the disease. When I need help or need help alone, feel sad or want to go out, I speak up. Saying it avoids any misunderstanding because they can't read my mind.

I leave the hospital, upset that I haven't had any of my favorite nurses in those three days. I am very emotional. It was already like this during my schooling, to please the teacher I tried to get good grades in his subject. This is what made me love French and hate math. It was also partly because the economics teacher was brilliant that I chose to do an economic and social bac.

After my first chemo, canker sores and mucositis appeared in my mouth. I looked for a natural solution to make my toothpaste myself. I ordered white clay which removes impurities, to this I add tea tree essential oil, which has an antiseptic effect, and liquid sodium bicarbonate, from the hospital, to form a paste. Since then I have had no problem with my mouth. Even the medical team were impressed. My oncologist validated the composition before I used it and I sent the recipe to her so that she can give it as needed. The nurse coordinator allows me to distribute it in the hospital, so I print out cards to put them in the waiting room. It is important to have your products validated, I have experienced this. At the start of my treatments, I was taking Desmodium in order to protect my liver. While I had asked for the essential oils, I did not find it useful to do so for the Desmodium, telling myself that it was a natural plant. When I listed my medications and supplements with the hospital pharmacist, he informed me that it could interact with one of my chemotherapy products. I stopped him immediately! The same problem also arises with St. John's Wort, which reduces the effectiveness of treatments.

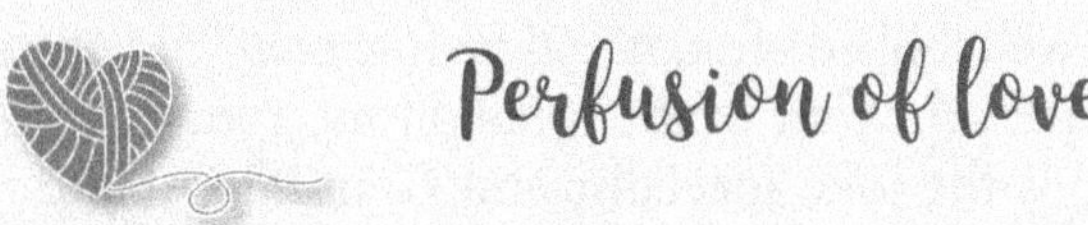

«Hello, I have printed your magic recipe and made it available to patients. I even gave it personally to some of them. Thank you again for this collective thought. Take care of you.»

In addition to the toothpaste, I went natural for my hair with goat milk shampoo. But right now I don't need it, shaved hair is super convenient! I save a lot of time not having to wash, dry and style them. Being hot, I feel lighter and besides, so funny, I have the same cut as my father-in-law. I hydrate my scalp with Even Cosmetics brand mist, their products are suitable for people in treatment. I love my bald head, it's okay to look at myself in the mirror. But I feel like I would «shock» if I went out without a turban.

Monday 13th August, as I am not doing too badly, unlike this weekend, and we have to plan everything at the last minute, we decide to go see my family who live 1 hour 30 minutes from Tours. My grandparents are happy to see me and although it is a tiring day, it is good.

Grandma accepts that I take off my turban.

- Ah, I expected worse. Looks good on you, even if you can tell you're sick, my poor darling.

In addition to seeing them less, I call them less often than before. Phone calls wear me out quickly, I have to concentrate and it ends up giving me a headache. My four grandparents are very attentive to the progress of the treatments. My grannies don't have the same temperament at all. There is one who says to me «This is unfair, why you, I do not understand» and the other who says «Come on! You will be well looked after, it will be fine now ". Despite their differences, the four of them taught me a lot. My grandpa Claude is the joke specialist and Grandma Aliette taught me how to bake my very first cake! My grandma Monique had the patience to teach me knitting and Grandpa Louis passed on his taste for writing to me.

My day 8, Thursday 16th August, marks my first time in an armchair room. I'm exhausted, I would have liked the calm of a single room with the comfort of a bed. There are four women in the room. Obviously, I am the youngest. The situation completely destabilizes me, I want to go home asap. It's dark, my large apple green armchair is fine, but it's positioned behind the front door of the room. The nurses and the doctors go back and forth incessantly to see the different patients. During this time, to make matters worse for the situation already beyond my control, mum and Flavien cannot stay with me, because the conversations are confidential. When the door finally closes, the lady in front of me asks me if it's okay.

- Not really, my red blood cells must be low, I feel so weak.

Speaking with her, I realize that it gives me a boost. She's getting ready to leave and I'm surprised she puts on a wig. I allow myself to point it out to him.

- I think your hair is fine.
- They are all gray and too short.

- This is the trend, young people have them discolored to make them gray.

She goes out laughing and wishing me good luck, but with her wig screwed on her head. It was a great meeting, in the end it's beneficial to be in a wheelchair.

The return home is difficult, I feel a great discomfort, I am terribly in pain. Luckily Flavien is there to help me, he puts on some music and I shower while sitting in the tub. These «fits» only last ten minutes, but it's intense and unsettling, I can feel them coming and I panic even more.

To forget this terrible news day I will move on by going to bed. But the night is not going any better, my bones are painful, my whole body is sore and I am in a cold sweat. I'm sick of it, the treatments have to end, I can't take it anymore! I did the hard part ... Normally. I'm afraid they'll give me hope for mild chemo, but my PET scan isn't good enough for it.

My blood test results are not good, I have 7.4 red blood cells, therefore a transfusion is scheduled for Sunday 19th August. What consoles me is that it will be in the blood department where I haven't been back since my first hospitalization for the announcement and I like this department and the medical team.

On the night of August 18-19, my buttocks hurt a lot, I spent a sleepless night trying to calm the pain by applying a lot of creams, taking a hot bath and then a cold. I twist in pain, I don't stay still, nothing relieves me. At 4 a.m. I call the blood department in utter desperation, but they won't allow me to come. I keep exploding with crying, screaming in pain, squealing like a little dog left alone all day. Flavien gives me a heating pad, then some ice cubes in a glove. He is helpless in front of my pain. I text the magnetizer I see sometimes, begging her to help me from a distance, but in the middle of the night she is asleep. Fortunately, I have an appointment at 9 am for my transfusion, but the wait is endless. The only thing you have to do is go to the emergency room in the other hospital in town. They won't do anything more to me, they don't know me… I'm staying at home, but I'm in pain.

From 8 o'clock, I go to the hematology department. One Sunday morning, it's quiet, I twist and scream in pain on the bedroom bed. Some caregivers know me and know that I am not exaggerating. We turn on the television to occupy my mind a bit and as a sign, the programmed channel is showing the music of *Bigflo and Oli* and their track *Demain*. I love these useful synchronicities at times like this.

«Don't think about it
Don't think about anything, nothing, nothing, nothing
It will be better tomorrow. «

The nurse finds me a buoy so that my buttocks are elevated. The doctor and the resident arrive at 10 am, my parents have arrived in the meantime. They explain to me that my blood test shows severe aplasia, the neutrophils are close to zero. My body no longer defends itself against aggression. My butt pain will get better when my white blood cells come back up, until they give me painkillers and antibiotics. The doctor decides to keep me for a few days, it is so painful that I prefer to stay in the hospital. What seems to worry them more than my pain is my low potassium level. Let's say potassium plays on the heart and it is best not to weaken it. At the end of the day, I have a fever and throw up what little food I managed to eat. The temperature only drops before I fall asleep.

To start the week, the nurse puts me on a morphine pump for 24 hours in small doses. On top of all of this, I have an ingrown toenail which hurts. I've had them regularly since I was little, but with the low number of white blood cells and platelets I can't seem to heal them without hurting myself further.

- I'm the queen of toe dolls! the nurse jokes.

She puts antiseptic on my toe and applies herself to wrapping the bandage. It is nice that the healthcare team takes the time to deal with ailments that might seem trivial, but which, if poorly treated, can quickly be painful. It's one less hassle! Another problem, out of control ... the gentleman from the next room spends his evenings on the phone and he has a very deep voice, it resonates. Hard to fall asleep, besides my pain.

When the night shift goes by around 4 o'clock, I can hardly wake up. A nurse can't think of anything better to do than lift my pajama top from the bottom to look at my PAC… PAC which sits above my chest! So I just have to pull my collar lightly like all the other nurses do and like I do most of the time. Too surprised to say anything and too drowsy to be upset, I fall back to sleep.

The next night, a nurse wants to remove my hydration because it is not noted in the prescriptions.

- What is this story ? No way you will remove my hydration, during all my hospitalizations it is the only one that is always connected!

- I have to ask the doctor on duty ... about hydration.

Mess ! Why are they so nasty at night? This time I won my case, I stay hydrated. The «pig's head» as my family called me when I was little… Ah, there! It serves my tenacity! To be honest, I don't think cancer could have happened on anyone other than me in my family, I'm the one who's most capable. Besides, I'd rather be in the action than watch helplessly a loved one go through all this shit. The professor on the ward has detected that I have character the few times he has seen me. He gently tells me that I know what I want. Besides, for me it's not a fault. It's important to be assertive, especially in the hospital I feel.

During the day, the nurses on the ward are more or less my age, it's nice to talk to them… Alizée is from 1994 like me. My favorite is Pauline! It makes me weird to see her, because she could clearly be a friend. There is also Jojo, a nursing assistant in her forties, who sets the mood in the ward. Tonight, she's offering me a scarf-tying class! She has brought pretty scarves, she ties two together to give volume and mix colors.

Looks like I'm starting to get better, certainly thanks to a strong painkiller that got me going for almost 3 hours, but at least I'm eating. I eat carbonara pasta, my safe bet that gives me morale.

It's already Friday, I've spent the week in the hospital, my white and red blood cells have come back up, but before I leave the hospital I have to see a specialist for my buttocks. For the first time, I get into an ambulance, because I am going to the other hospital in Tours. The specialist tells me that these are cracks, I have to apply a cream and do Dakin baths. He also informs me that ultra-yeast diarrhea is dangerous when you have PAC. Has anyone found it interesting to report this to me before?

A few days of respite, even if I quickly exhaust myself, with Flavien we go out for a walk. A boat trip on the Vienne, a visit to the Sleeping Beauty castle in Ussé, a visit to Vouvray and a tavern with friends. I have very few days when I'm fine, when I do we try to take the opportunity to see friends and family as we often have to turn down invitations.

Hard prick

"I didn't invite you, I knew you couldn't."

I should have started my fifth cycle of BEACOPP, but today, Wednesday August 29th is PET Scan day! If this one is good, tomorrow I will have milder chemo; ABVD. Flavien accompanies me and then we take refuge in Feuillette to devour their bacon strings!

The next day, the doctor arrives in my room:

- So, are you happy?
- Sorry ? Happy with what? I missed something.
- We go to ABVD!

The same doctor explained the results of the second PET scan to me. She is not my referring doctor. The professor told me that they were going to work together to make the decision and there the doctor seems to be making the decision on her own ... We ask to see the professor on the ward to be sure of the protocol. He takes the time to explain it to me.

- Are you on a plane, do you let yourself be transported or do you go to the cockpit?
- Ah bah! If I have the chance, of course I'll see how it goes at the controls!
- Ahah, I recognize you there! But don't worry, we're switching to the ABVD protocol. There's almost nothing left, we're not going to hurt you any more.

Immediate take-off, direction four pockets. One of 15 minutes, the second of 30 minutes, the third of 15 minutes and the fourth and last of 2:30. We do not forget the rinse product of a few minutes between the bags and the premedication, namely seven tablets of cortisone and an antinausea drug. The cool thing about this change in protocol is that I'm sleeping at home tonight! It's only one day in the day hospital every two weeks. It feels good to sleep at home, but where is the lady who asks me «What can I get you for breakfast?» «Where's my breakfast in bed? The scam!

Indeed, the ABVD seems less violent, I slept well for that first night after treatment. However, its share of side effects didn't forget to bother me. My cheeks are red and hot with cortisone. I feel sprayed non-stop, I have stomach cramps, but I have an appetite. When the appetite is good, is everything okay? At home, this is totally true! Eating is a real pleasure and when the taste goes, my morale takes a hit. I have specific food cravings. I eat all the variations of potatoes: mash, dauphine potatoes, pancakes, sautéed potatoes, not to mention the fries!

Tomorrow is the first day of school ! Flavien will do his first day as a mechanical engineer in a company north of Tours. Mum is back to work and Dad is going to have to take care of his own during the day since he has been retired since the start of the summer. The last few months I've been surrounded by lots of people, it's going to be a big change of pace for me and for Flavien. We made the decision to change rentals and look for a maisonette, because my 40 m2 apartment is extremely poorly insulated, in the summer it is way too hot and the winter way too cold. We had an appointment with Citya, the agency through which I currently rent my apartment. We would like to visit two accommodations.

- I remember you ! the salesperson assures me.

The salesperson never called back. That's why I'm calling Orpi.

- Hello, we are looking for a rental with two bedrooms north of Tours.

[…]

- I am on sick leave, but with daily allowances and my companion is on a permanent contract.

- Why sick leave?

- Cancer.

- Ah, but we're not going to have anything for you at all! Thank you goodbye.

Our research is off to a good start ...

September 15th is World Lymphoma Day. A week before, the hospital is organizing a conference on the subject. Mum is with me. There are around 100 men and women of all ages in the medical school amphitheater next to the hospital. For two hours, we learned a lot about lymphoma in general. Hodgkin has received little attention because he is poorly represented in the statistics. I saw the professionalism of the doctor, whom I had little confidence in, so I am reviewing my judgment.

A few days later, I take the bus for the first time in a long time. It moves a lot. It's a bad idea that I'm starting to regret very much. After 20 minutes, I arrive in town where I join Noémie, Deborah and Blandine for a snack. I had not seen Noémie since she was in the hospital for my first treatment. We talk to each other less and to put it mildly. Blandine and Deborah are nurses, in addition to understanding technical terms, I feel they are less embarrassed to talk about cancer. It's nice. Noémie hides the fact that I have no more hair and automatically comes to me asking for a clip or a rubber band for her hair. I'll laugh about it, but later. To save me the inconvenience of the bus, Flavien comes to pick me up in town.

On Wednesday September 13th, it's my dad who takes me for my second chemo of the fifth cycle. Yesterday I spent my day depressed and crying because I thought I was ugly. It's not easy everyday to accept yourself bald and your face swollen from the drugs. Arriving at the hospital, I meet the lady who was in front of me, in the ward with the chairs, but this time… without a wig! We address a knowing smile. I'm proud of myself if my comment may have helped her come to terms in part. I'm in a wheelchair so dad can't stay with me, he's waiting in the common room… from 10 am to 4 pm. Usually the sessions are held in silence, but now the ladies who are with me are chatty.

- Oh no, but for me it is essential that I keep a professional activity I cannot stay at home doing nothing.

None of us three answers. I wonder, because in my case, running a coffee in the morning is my most sporting activity of the day. To find out more, I ask my little Instagram community the question: «Did you continue to work during your cancer?» thanks to a «Yes» or «No» voting function, the result is undeniable, only 10% continued to work during the treatments. It really depends on the protocols, but as a general rule these are heavy treatments, hardly compatible with the work. I come out of the hospital tired, but painless.

This weekend, the exhibition fair is organized in my hometown, Loudun. I lived there from my 3 to 18 years old and my parents still live there. I did all my schooling there, inevitably I meet a lot of people I know. Many look away from me and some have no choice but to stop when we come face to face. They feel so uncomfortable! Not me. Ah, sacred taboo disease!

I am sad and disappointed, I expected my girlfriend Noémie to be more present for me. Since the start of the treatments we have only seen each other twice, I had few messages and they were awkward. I know I can tell her anything and since it has been eating me up for weeks I send her a message. She tells me she didn't realize it. Her return to France, after a year in the United States, unsettled her and she did not want to complain about «so little» in relation to my illness. I talk a lot about cancer because it is my daily life, but I can totally hear the concerns and other concerns of those around me. Especially since I understand his blues which I also felt when I came back from Ireland. I hope that trading will improve things between us.

I just passed 1000 followers on Instagram. «This might be a detail for you, but for me it means a lot, it means ...» What does it mean? Is it because I'm sick that more people are following me today or is it my blog writing job and my involvement in taking great photos that interests them?

Thursday 20th September, I do the tests for my breath, then an ultrasound of the heart to check that everything is fine. These exams are recurrent, in addition to the electrocardiograms performed during my hospitalizations. But this time the cardiologist is pushing the probe so hard on my chest that it hurts! As we are in the hospital, I take the opportunity to see the psychologist, an appointment that lasts barely an hour. I always feel like I have to hurry when I talk to him, I feel rushed. Dad, who accompanied me to the meetings, drops me off at the tavern to meet up with my blogging friends from Tours. The music is too loud, it makes an unpleasant hubbub. I have a hard time hearing girls so Flavien quickly comes to pick me up after work. This weekend, he is going to the Lot to join his friends. From my side, it will be a little quieter; with my parents, we eat in the restaurant and they take me to attend a sewing class, given by the tissus shop. This is the first time that I have done an activity in a group. A woman looks at me insistently, I approach her.

- Are you telling me something, but I don't know where?
- Hematology, she answers me softly, approaching.
- Oh yes ! Anyway, it couldn't be anywhere else, I haven't been going out much in recent months.

A pleasant moment of sewing to make a tote bag, it gives me morale.

For the past month, every Tuesday afternoon, mum has come to clean the apartment. I'm not fit enough to do this and Flavien is already doing a lot in addition to his job. Since it's a fit day, I ask him to take me to *Zodio* store to prepare for the creative workshop that I will be leading on 13th October. The store team seems excited about my idea for a star origami light garland.

A few days after my penultimate chemo, I cry from fatigue. I'm not doing anything, I'm not getting anywhere. It's a roller coaster ride, because in a few hours I can go from "good" to very bad. I watch the neighbors' cute cat lounging on the deckchair. He is a beautiful gray Maine Coon so he has long hair and a lion's head. If I'm in good shape, I call him and he comes to my door for a hug. Since I lost my Siamese, Chanelle, in December 2016, I have dreamed of adopting a new cat. It was very difficult for me to recover from his disappearance. When I saw the psychologist at the hospital at the start of treatment, I only talked about this. I even wondered if my sadness could be the cause of my lymphoma. At the moment in an apartment, it is not the ideal place and the doctors have clearly advised me against it with the treatment which weakens my immune system and therefore increases the risk of infection.

6th October is National Caregiver Day. The entourage often powerless, but ready for anything! Six months since the treatments have started, yet they continue to face and move forward with me while managing their own emotions in addition to mine. It is a physically and psychologically draining ordeal. My parents, my in-laws, but also, on the front line, my boyfriend. He did not run away and put aside his plans and desires. He has to do almost everything, shopping, eating, often helping me get dressed, sometimes washing me. He's the one who manages the medications I need to take. He comforts me, and much more ... and much worse ... Thank you, Flavien, for being my caregiver whom I love so much.

We're going to see Lucas, Flavien's nephew who just turned two. Once again, he refuses to give me a kiss. I wonder if it's because of the turban, I'm a little upset because he kindly said hello to Uncle Flavien. I console myself by telling myself that most of the little ones refuse to say hello and we always force them to kiss even though I don't like this very French custom.

October 11th is my last chemo !!!!

Chemo advices

Little recap to go in chemo serenely:

- ☐ Put on my patch
- ☐ Take a blanket
- ☐ Syrup to drink more water
- ☐ My colorful tablecloth
- ☐ Peppermint candies
- ☐ The notebook with my questions
- ☐ A book to wait

I am torn between joy and sadness, several feelings come over me. I'm in a wheelchair for the last one, but mum and dad are by my side. In some hospitals, the medical staff are ringing a bell for the latest chemo drugs. Nothing is set up here so my parents ring a bell on the phone right before I am unplugged. Immediately after my last chemo session, I see the psychologist at the hospital to share my conflicting feelings. I am reassured that she will continue to follow me even though I no longer have treatment. I'm afraid of what's next and I'm sad the chemo is over. I shouldn't be thinking this! In the hospital, I'm in a cocoon and now I'm afraid of the unknown. I feel kicked off the plane, heading into an unknown jungle.

I received a shower of hearts! A nice idea from mum who sent wooden hearts to my loved ones asking to personalize them and then mail them to me. I got so many! For example Boris and his family, from Bordeaux, who regularly hear from me. There is even my Irish family! And my former chef from Bordeaux! Too strong !

The chemos are therefore over! We will have to wait until the beginning of December to hear the word remission.

In the meantime, what do I do?

Booster injection

The hard times of pain are over. The still present fatigue will subside. When I think of the fact that I have supported "I had cancer" all my life, it turns my head. This is completely crazy !

Two days after my last chemo, I have a big day related to my blog. I lead a creative workshop at Zodio in Tours on the occasion of "Blogging Day" organized by the store. I am touched, because Julie, one of the bloggers, suggested that everyone put on a turban so that I am not the only one wearing one. Some of the girls played along, but also many vendors. We are a dozen bloggers to lead workshops throughout the day. My workshop is at 4 pm to give me time to come home and take a nap just before. Exhausting, but with the help of Flavien, I took my workshop to the end.

To change from the hospital, we leave for five days on the Ile de Ré. I am weak and can do little, but I have been loaned a wheelchair and I plan to enjoy the sea air anyway. The laboratory calls me and informs me that my red blood cell count is low and that I am contacting the hospital. I call my hematologist and negotiate a new blood test. But when I get back, I have 7.7 red blood cells, that means I'm going to have another transfusion.

- Come on, let's go to the hospital!

I arrive at 10 a.m. but at noon the nurse explains to me, while taking my blood through the PAC, that the blood test was not signed by the Loudun laboratory, that it is therefore not validated. It takes two hours for a complete, signed and validated blood formulation. The blood bags are coming, it's 4 p.m.! Dad left to donate blood. It's the first time, I'm very proud of him. He was afraid of needles and blood tests, but he overcomes his apprehension because he knows how important it is. At 6.30 p.m., the caregiver offers me the meal tray:

- Keep your tray, me tonight, I eat chestnuts! I explain with enthusiasm.

I love wood-fired chestnuts. Titi and Gigi went to great lengths to prepare everything well. Thierry, whom I call Titi, is a colleague of daddy who has always been there for me. He has a role of godfather. I'm enjoying myself, but I'm exhausted and unfortunately I have to cut the evening short.

Already a month since the chemos are finished. My nails are streaked. I see four white lines on each nail, four like the number of BEACOPP I received. For years, my nails have been long and strong, it pains me to see them so brittle even though I have always protected them with nail polish. But what worries me are the red patches that are reappearing around my eyes and in my mouth, the same as before my diagnosis. I have also had pain in my shoulder for no reason for several weeks. My referring doctor at the hospital is giving me a chest x-ray. She can't see anything, it calms me a bit.

The blood tests are spaced every two weeks. I continue to take my medications, antivirals and antibacterials until my immune system returns to normal, because the white blood cells are still poor. I have four pills to take every day, plus another every other day, the huge Bactrim, which I regularly choke on.

To get back in shape, I start yoga. These are free classes offered at the hospital. I've never been athletic so in addition to giving myself a quiet moment, yoga works my whole body gently. Dad takes me out every Monday because I haven't resumed driving. I would be dangerous on the road, I don't have enough reflexes and I don't know the distance. I haven't been driving since the beginning of April, that is to say before the diagnosis.

Despite the exhaustion, I want to stay active, write, tinker, move... but I am held back because my heart is racing and my legs are shaking. These short attempts at activity quickly end lying on the couch resting in front of a series. The treatments have been causing me cognitive impairment for the past few months. When I am tired, I easily let go of my cutlery and above all I lose my words. Used to speaking fast and a lot, I am in slow motion. The microwave becomes a fridge, the sink a sink, and a hot-air balloon becomes a wind helicopter. I play guessing games with Flavien. To make it easier for him, I remain in the lexical field of my word.

A few months ago, La Roche-Posay contacted the bloggers of Tours to offer a discovery day. Mainly interested in the post-cancer cure, I replied to the email explaining my situation. We therefore agreed to create a group of "Kfighters" to come and discover the treatments adapted to our needs. I naturally proposed to the Kopines with whom I chat on Instagram: Alice, a Belgian who was diagnosed with Hodgkin a month and a half before me. Jennifer, diagnosed with b lymphoma a few days before me. Alison, diagnosed with Hodgkin's lymphoma the same day as me with the same stage and the same treatments. Laura, who has also had Hodgkin since February. Gladys, being treated for breast cancer. Nour, who I've never spoken to, but who seems bubbly through her Instagram where she shares her journey of caring for ovarian cancer. And with one spot remaining, Jennifer asks if Coralie can join us, as she is the one she has the most in common with her cancer.

On November 8 and 9, we therefore left every eight for 24 hours to discover the thermal baths of La Roche-Posay. Dad is taking me, it's 1 hour 30 minutes from Loudun. On the road, I suddenly don't want to go. I dread being around people for 24 hours. Finally, I want to be alone on my couch. It doesn't sound like me. I'm more of the type who enjoys meeting new people, especially since I've been getting to know girls on social media for months! We arrive one after the other at the end of the afternoon at the hotel where we are kindly lodged for the night. We gather in one of the bedrooms. It is both unsettling and interesting to meet women who have been through almost the same things at the same time. Jennifer and Coralie are just coming out of an autologous bone marrow transplant, they seem to be in good shape, I am impressed.

After a good night's sleep, we join Lydie, web manager, who is waiting for us at the Pavillon Rose, a place dedicated to people touched by cancer. The La Roche-Posay cure is aimed at all cancers, but specializes in breast cancer. Many curists are present for skin problems such as psoriasis, burns, eczema of the child… We visit the thermal baths and after the meal, we are entitled to a moment of relaxation in the spa which is independent of the thermal baths and therefore open to all. I'm surprised they're all in good spirits. I am in the difficult «after» phase where I constantly want to cry when for six months I kept smiling and was positive. I am reflecting an image that is not really mine, but I find it difficult to hide my low morale. The girls seem happy, I feel guilty for reacting like that. Afterwards I completely destabilize myself, I feel lost. I am withdrawn and sad. We are not told that after treatment is difficult to manage and those around us do not understand.

Three weeks later, I take the train to go to the big craft fair in Paris. I got up early to meet Charlotte, a blogger from Tours who also goes to this event. I dread this day again. Before I would have been enthusiastic, this is a great event that I am attending for the first time. I am stressed that I don't have time to do everything, to be tired, to have pain in my foot… Fortunately, Charlotte guides me out of the train to easily reach the exhibition center. I find Nour and Alison, we are delighted to see each other again and spend the day together. With Alison, we make Nour discover many creative hobbies, she wants to try everything. They are happy, energetic, they make me laugh, it's nice to spend the day with them. At the show, I meet an Instagramer I met at *Zodio* last month. She's creative and funny ... Maybe a little too funny, she forces the joke. She shows us a nice stand that she is going to go to and invites us to come by, which we do a few minutes later. When we approach the booth, she introduces us in a ... special way.

- This is the cancer team, they are happy to be alive!

I smile, but I am completely sawed off by his indelicacy. Nour and Alison have their eyes going out of their sockets, they move away immediately. I say a few words, but it's the fog in my head. I quickly join the girls who are stunned by his behavior. Among ourselves, we laugh easily about the disease, but when it's someone totally outside, who we hardly know, it can be out of place and very upsetting. They are amazed when I tell them that she made the same kind of remark to me a few weeks ago at Zodio. Telling myself that cancer is a good excuse not to fuck around at home and let my boyfriend do it all. A few days later, we explain our way of thinking to him by message.

Thursday 22nd November, I have a classic CT scan with the prior injection of a contrast product and on 27 th November, good news, no more traces of the disease on my CT scan: complete answer!

When I announced my cancer, I realized the small indelicacies committed by the people I spoke to. I've had all kinds of reactions, from the most neutral to the most shocked, even shocking to me. It is not easy to find the right words if a loved one announces their illness to you. Words can be lacking when we are faced with an ad that upsets our enthusiasm for life. I'm sure I was the first one to be awkward with those around me when something big happened in their life. Therefore, I decided to publish on my blog an article «How to deal with the illness of a loved one? «

1 - Do not remain silent.

You learned of the illness from someone you haven't heard from for a long time. If this person has mattered at some point in your life, don't be silent. A letter, a short message can do a lot of good. It's okay not to know what to say, feel free to express it or just send «I'm thinking of you». For example, my uncle regularly sends me a heart of a different color. I have received messages from people I haven't heard from in 10 years. It warmed my heart.

2 - Avoid comparing ... «I know someone who ...»

I have noticed that we tend to relate to a known situation. Either because we don't know what to say or because we think we are comforting the person. For the first few days after the announcement, I wanted to be listened to, to talk about my situation. I still didn't realize and couldn't pronounce the word cancer. I didn't want to hear that neighbor Germaine, 70 years old and three cancers, was living very well between two chemo's with all her hair on her head. Every disease is different! Each patient is different! It is not comparable depending on the progress of the disease, the age, the philosophy of the person.

3 - Avoid dramatizing.

The people around me were more afraid than me. It was in their words or looks that I understood the importance of what was falling on me. The panic messages brought me back to reality.

4 - «Keep me informed!»
This sentence I have received dozens of times. Sometimes I feel like talking, sometimes I don't, but one thing's for sure I'm not going to send a message or phone everyone around me to let them know one by one about the progress. Without actually receiving messages every other day, I appreciated that friends tell me they will hear from me. It changes everything! Especially when they really do.

5 - Do not hesitate to question.
You can ask if the person wants to talk about it. Asking questions is the only way to know. «Do you want a visit? «When can I go by without disturbing you?» Here are some suitable questions. Some treatments are cumbersome and make visits complicated, if not sometimes impossible, with fatigue, falling white blood cells and the risk of infection. If you want to help, offer concrete things other than «Don't hesitate if you need to». For example, vegetables from the garden, a drive to the hospital, the loan of a book ...

While being careful with what you say, the important thing is to be yourself and be sincere in your reaction.

The weekends are definitely busy, this weekend is the Flavien engineering school gala in Tarbes. Lots of road, but which passes quickly with two people by carpooling. At noon, it is the «family» meal at his school, the atmosphere is warm. I did not know at all the concept of «families» according to affinities in higher schools. In the evening, during his class meal, I allow myself my first drink of alcohol since the announcement of cancer. Rosé, although I prefer white wine. After the meal, we head to the venue for the gala. We wait a long time, outside, in the cold, before entering the huge hall that will accommodate more than three thousand people. The decoration is magnificent on the theme of the odyssey of the seabed. But I have to sit down quickly, the deafening music turns my head.

- Why do you have that on your head? asks a fifty-something, pointing to my turban.

Neither one nor two I take off my turban and let my bald head appear.

- Okay, that's okay! he said to me, shrugging his shoulders.

A few minutes later, two young people approach me. I hear badly, one of the two young people shows me my turban. I go to take it off, he nods no and comes up to my ear to explain.

- My friend found a scarf on the floor and he wants to tie it on his head, can you help him?

I find the process fun and apply myself to making my favorite knot. It just goes to show that age does not mean anything about whether or not you are comfortable with the disease. They go back to dance, delighted with this headgear.

Today 11th December, I have a mission: to get my doctor off the ground! But she is slow in her explanations.

- So I'm in remission?
- You could say that. But there is a «scar» and you don't know what's going on underneath.

Yeah well ... she didn't say it, but it's just like! I am in remission! You have to, the Kopines are, why not me? I take this opportunity of coming to the hospital to thank the medical team from both departments who treated me. I'm bringing two boxes of chocolates, candies, and some funny syringe-shaped pens.

During my treatments in June, with the help of the hospital social worker, I applied for a disabled parking card and just received it. Obviously, I would have preferred to use it during my treatments, but it will come in handy when I go back to driving. I absolutely have to drive again, because on February 11 I am participating in the Salon des Trends Créatives in Tours. With a few bloggers from Tours, we have a stand to offer creative workshops for four days.

Kristen, my American girlfriend, celebrates Christmas in Paris and comes to Tours for a day. I thus meet her boyfriend, Michael, and she with Flavien. Kristen, I met her in 2013 while studying in Tours. In addition to a physical resemblance, we have a lot in common. I am happy to see her again and to introduce them to Breton pancakes… in Tours!

With Flavien, we have nothing planned for the New Year and luckily, because I can't get over my fatigue from family meals for Christmas. Christmas was special, it's like I was disconnected, I didn't feel like I was there. I couldn't bend down at the foot of the tree to open the presents and I had to go to bed early. For the 31st, we bought gourmet dishes at Picard, we are going to spend a beautiful evening quietly and too bad if we fall asleep before midnight! My cousin has often said to me:

- You're not taking advantage of your youth Laura!

But after this ordeal, I am convinced that enjoying life is not about partying every night. For me, enjoying life is traveling to discover a different culture or a new corner of France with Flavien. Enjoying is also making me happy by going to a restaurant or doing creative hobbies.

At the start of 2019, I am 25 years old, have 25 hairs on my head and I am in remission! Yeah! I have much less hair than when I was born and as often on my birthday,

I'm sick! My birthday present is to go to an unknown destination for the weekend. Flavien organized, prepared and paid for everything.

- Love the idea! What am I taking?

Quick, quick, after his day's work we rush to the station and I discover that we are leaving for Lille! A city that I have really wanted to visit for a while. By train, this is done rather quickly. It's beautiful, we make the most of the weekend, we eat fat local specialties, but delicious. Glad to see that I am fit enough to travel again, I didn't think I could.

Only a few days after our return, I am very ill and that scares me. Not all the bacteria lying around on the trains must have improved my condition. I call the SAMU who advises me to go to the emergency room given my history. It is already 11:30 p.m. when I arrive in the emergency room at the clinic next to my house. There is nobody, everything is calm. I was quickly put into a cubicle, but I waited forever to see a doctor. My parents are arriving to replace Flavien who is working tomorrow morning. I get home at 5:30 am, they just rehydrated me and took a blood test, but I'm relieved, I'm okay with nothing. Simply gastroenteritis.

To end this month of January well, we are recovering the keys to our new rental. A small house with a garden on the street next to the apartment! With two bedrooms, I will be able to set up my dreamy creative workshop. In order to adopt a cat, alerts from surrounding associations are already all activated. Our parents are helping us to move, close to the apartment, the installation is quick. I am of no use, because too weak. It makes me sad to watch the apartment empty, I felt good in it even though it is poorly insulated and there is no possibility of having internet.

We can finally plan beyond the next day, so we plan getaways of a few days. The next will be in Normandy! And with all the bridges in May, we would like to go south to Rodez to discover the area and see Carine, Flavien's cousin. I'm into decorating the house, we agreed on duck blue.

If I get ahead on everything, I feel like I'm stagnating with the psychologist at the hospital. So I consult that of the IETO37 association, a support network for cancer patients in the Center region. I explain to him my anger towards people in general and my resentment towards those who have not shown any signs of life since the announcement of my cancer. Thanks to my exchanges with her, I better understand the different reactions. Cancer is frightening, people are afraid of death and being sick and to protect themselves they do not talk about it. If we don't talk about it, it doesn't exist! It's time to de-stigmatize cancer!

Hard prick

"I wasn't really around you but I couldn't handle having someone I might lose when I wasn't sure I would continue on my own."

I have been driving alone again for a few days now, it was about time as I start the four day marathon at the Creative Leisure Show. It's going to be great, I have several workshops planned, but not too early, because in the morning I struggle to prepare. Once there, I'm afraid of not having anyone in my workshops, I take care of my hands by demonstrating modeling with cold *Cleopatre* porcelain.

«I'm here to see what he's doing, the young man,» a lady said to me as she approached the booth before correcting her words.

I am so upset! My blogger friends comfort me, but tomorrow I'm putting on earrings! And a dress! No but !

I was held on to the adrenaline rush, but after four days on the living room, I collapse on the couch and won't move for at least a week. I am exhausted, but delighted with this experience. The workshops were very popular and I loved presenting and sharing my different passions.

- Monday 19th February, here are the headlines: death of Karl Lagerfeld in the American hospital in Paris following a long illness ...

I don't give the presenter time to finish ...

- Ah! They annoy me with their «long illness» it's always like that. We guess, but we do not say the word cancer! It's not going to become less taboo with journalists!

The time has come for my first haircut, they grow back ash blonde and very thin, but without holes. I make an appointment with my hairdresser. I met Line at the end of my treatments, she opened this summer and is one of the few Tours lounges that are partners of the Solid'Hair association. I congratulated him and we talked and hit it off. A few months ago she gave me a scalp massage which stimulated the regrowth of my hair and it was a very pleasant moment. She is comfortable with the illness, it makes conversation easier. As I don't really enjoy going to the hairdresser, I really feel like I'm at a friend's house who is having tea.

I'm going to get my hair done for the photo shoot offered to me by Delphine, a photographer I met on Instagram.

But first, I have an appointment with the allergist, to solve the mystery of my red patches on my face and especially on my neck. She puts 152 patches, yes 152, on my back on Monday and I have to come back on Wednesday and Friday to see the progress. At the end of the week, she notices that I am allergic to fragrances: perfumes, spray, misters ... Mainly scents of flowers such as lily of the valley, jasmine, mimosa ... Once at home, I realize that the barbaric names are present in many beauty and maintenance products.

I attend a support group organized by the IETO37 association and led by two psychologists. I am with five other women, mainly suffering from breast cancer. Many things are in place for these women, communication on the subject is important since two out of eight women are concerned in France. The talk groups are enriching, but the women, mainly retired, do not have the same issues as me. "Will I find a job after cancer? «» Will the bank give me a mortgage? «

For the control of the three months of remission, since the announcement in December, I have had a classic CT scan with a contrast agent. I know this exam well, I have taken it several times. But this time, I stay in the machine for a long time and when I should have gone out, they inject me with the contrast agent a second time. I am in tears when I stand up from the exam table. The student who gave me the IV is missing. The nurse is taking care of me and he tries to talk to me about other things, but I get back to what I'm here for.

- I can't tell you anything, the nurse explains.

... That says it all. I know it.

The verdict was not long in coming since on 6th March I have an appointment with my doctor, I am accompanied by dad, it is the eve of his birthday.

I'll have to start over, go back.

My check-up scan is not good, the disease is returning.

I thought it was all behind me and at the same time I suspected it. I felt that it was not all over. Plus on Sunday I started coughing again. A very peculiar cough that drums in my left lung.

I'm sad and angry, I'm scared. This time, I blame the whole world! I envy the apparent levity of the people I meet in the street.

- I don't want to be in the percentage who die from it.

Signalling error

After three days of confusion, I get over the news. Words fail me to express what I feel, I receive several positive messages, nicely worded. For cancer which, in most cases, can be cured in six months… It will take longer than expected.

The previous two weekends, we had a meal with our families and this evening we had to welcome our friends to celebrate my 25 years, the remission and the move. We do not have the strength to prepare the planned aperitif dinner. We invited them to spend the afternoon more spaced out, to make it quieter. In the meantime, this morning, we join Flavien's cousin, Grégory and his girlfriend Manon at a wellness salon south of Tours. It is good that Manon told me about this salon, I am intrigued by a conference entitled «Learning how to heal». A solar woman, dressed in a long yellow dress welcomes us. His words are sweet and resonate with me. I end the conference with tears in my eyes. We are about to leave, but ...

- Maybe I should have asked her what exactly she does for care and where she is, I say to Manon.

Neither one nor two, Manon is leading me on the stand. I learn that Christelle does energy healing, in particular Reiki, and that she lives only five minutes from my house. I really want to give it a try so I make an appointment. I am glad.

Manon and Grégory join us at home, followed by a few friends, it's good to see them, even if the mood is no longer at the party. I take this opportunity to send a message to Anthony who wasn't present during the first treatments.

He is a very good friend that I met during my studies six years ago. We confided in each other a lot and because of his personal history he has a hard time with the disease ... but I need support! Let him show me he's here!

Despite this news that brings us down, we have not canceled our weekend in Normandy with Flavien. Discovering the coast, it changes our ideas. We join Noémie in Rouen, where she is studying. Before returning to Touraine, we had a brunch with a friend from the summer camp, Émilie.

A very pleasant weekend, but it's already Monday and I'm back in the hospital to take another biopsy. After waiting three hours for the radiologist, Flavien goes to look for a McDonalds that we eat in the oncology hall with dad! I didn't want the meal tray so I savored this moment that was not in keeping with the habits of such a place. The hospital is downtown, the nurses explained to me that I could have whatever I wanted delivered to me. The medical team orders regularly, but also many patients, as the food in the hospital can quickly become disgusting. This is the most unusual place where I have eaten McDonalds.

On Tuesday 19th March, my biopsy is performed very early. Without general anesthesia, the puncture of the lung will be painful. The team settles me in, I am worried, but quickly reassured, because the hypnotherapist comes to join me. Until the last minute, no one was able to tell me if she would be present. Fortunately, she is by my side. I close my eyes and she sends me off to a fantasy world while the doctors bustle around me. After several passages in the scanner to locate the only accessible mass, they plant a needle of two millimeters which is a kind of straw. I smell slightly, it's unpleasant, but sustainable. Back in my room I have a pain in my chest. Certainly the tissues «upset» by the procedure. Hours go by and the medics force me to lie down. Without further explanation, I pass a radio without leaving my room. I didn't even know it was possible! I am slightly upright, my back hurts. It's only in the evening that my doctor finally arrives.

- It's normal for you to have pain, it's a pneumothorax. The membrane around the lung has come off, there is air all around. Don't get up, it will subside within 24 hours.

Indeed, the next day I am better, I can go home. In the mailbox, my little monthly happiness awaits me, the Pause Moderne box. Each month's theme is an adjective and this month it totally fits me, because I'm going to have to be: CONFIDENT. Inside is a «Confident, Happy, Sexy» card, treats, a self-confidence booklet and most importantly an embroidery kit. I discovered embroidery in Ireland where my host family introduced me. Since then I hadn't taken the time to equip myself so I am going immediately.

The weekend promises to be beautiful, Flavien gave me roses and a good breakfast to inaugurate our new garden room. In the afternoon, I watch him plant our first crops. I would like to take care of our little garden, but I have to keep off touching the ground and I am weak, I have a hard time squatting. I'm still less exhausted than I was a few weeks ago. A «new life» is how the psychologist describes this sudden energy that I had lost.

Tuesday 26th March, I have an appointment with my doctor. The samples confirm that it is still Hodgkin's disease. It's already that ! It happens that there are cells of another type of lymphoma. I will have three or four chemotherapy treatments followed by an autologous transplant with a stay in the sterile room for at least three weeks. The chemo is called R-DHAP. Still a bunch of drugs with unpronounceable names that all aim to hit my cells hard without exception. I was expecting this treatment or the ICE protocol because I spoke to the girls who had relapsed on Instagram. I also spoke with Coralie, Jennifer and Fanny who had an autologous transplant for B lymphoma. They all had reassuring words.

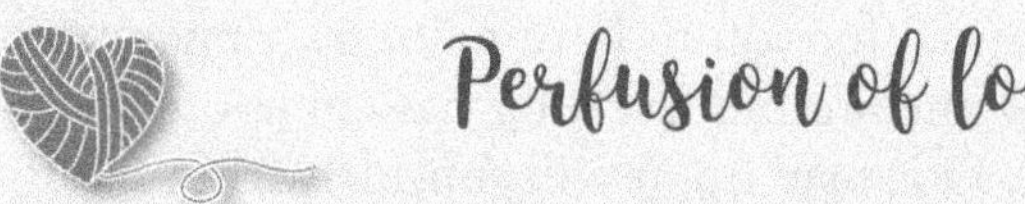

"What the disease taught me and which has become my mantra: you experience the negative and you create the positive! We understood that if we didn't move around to experience cool stuff, it didn't happen by itself!»

I'm not really into a relapse because the cancer cells came back less than six months after the treatments were finished. I am resistant to the first line of treatment. I know what to expect, on the one hand it's good, I'm prepared, but on the other hand it freaks me out because the treatments are going to be different. Certainly more violent for my weakened body. This time, I got ready, I ordered a multicolored pillbox, essential for navigating through all the medications.

I'm starting the new protocol on 9th April, before we go to the Hoshi concert. It's one of Mum and Dad's Christmas presents. This concert comes at the right time, just before the resumption of chemo. Hoshi's melodies helped me a lot during the first treatments, the concert will boost me.

Thanks to my mutual health insurance, I called in a cleaning lady to relieve mom. I dread a lot and it keeps me awake. It's not easy to leave your house to a stranger, even though I'm here. It will never be done like me or mom. I'm worried that she might not adhere to the natural products I use for the household. I'm afraid she'll put too much scent on her and end up with a headache for the rest of the day. I dread having to hold a conversation with her and being exhausted. But… it's going well! She is used to using white vinegar and she even gives me advice. She's low-key and my house is spotless in just two hours. Tomorrow afternoon, mum will come and we can go do some shopping, take the time to chat without her rushing to do the housework. I am entitled to this help four times because my health insurance does not consider my relapse to be «serious enough». I should be hospitalized for at least fifteen consecutive days to extend the household help!

I see Christelle for a Reiki session. I explain to her that I dread the return to the hospital, the meal trays, the smells, the depressing colors of the premises... She advises me to bring a colored tablecloth to put on the bedroom table. Maybe it can help me eat. She also recommends that I view hospital food as something that will nourish me, give me strength, and not to make me happy. After massages, the session ends with an assessment of my feelings and I draw, at random, an oracle card which gives me a positive message in connection with my worries of the moment.

I have an appointment at 3 p.m. in hematology. I am stressed and want to cry. When it's over, we forget, we take advantage and when we have to go back it is by throwing up everything that we do not have in the stomach, it is so difficult. To change my mind, mum invites me to the restaurant. Next door, the juice bar is open so I have a drink for the hospital. Installed in my room, I unfold my multicolored polka-dot tablecloth, I put down my colorful magazine and my raspberry-banana smoothie. I'm happy with myself, it's colorful, it makes me happy. As soon as we arrive, an intern tells me that it will be DHAP chemo and not R-DHAP and that I will be staying in the hospital for three days when I thought I would stay two days. The first product is on 24 hours and I'm going to have four days of cortisone. It's going to be nice for Flavien at home, the cortisone gets on my nerves and makes me unpleasant. It's 6 p.m., I'm still waiting for the first product, the wait is long, my head hurts, I'm torturing my mind. What if DHAP was as hard to bear as BEACOPP? Plus, I forgot to put the EMLA numbing patch on my PAC. We quickly lose the habit. Above all, I am very head in the air. At 6:30 p.m. the nurse comes to my room.

- Before starting chemo, we need to test your kidneys. For six hours, we will pass pockets of water.

I panic, I don't see myself alone in the middle of the night if I react badly to the product. The memory of the first difficult nights with BEACOPP haunts me. Luckily, mum has her things planned for sleeping in the hospital that night, even though she's working tomorrow. While waiting for midnight, my trips to the bathroom are incalculable. The night nurse puts down the first bag and stays with us for twenty minutes to make sure no problems arise. I go back to sleep until 4 a.m., constant check time. The night is going well, I am stunned, but I am not in pain.

This midday, it is too late for me to choose my meal, but the caregiver offers me a kind of couscous and fries. French fries are always a pleasure! After an hour long nap, mum and dad arrive. But I'm tired, I don't really want to talk. I should have told them not to come, because they're still an hour's drive from the hospital! At 4 p.m. I see the psychologist at the hospital.

The chemo the second night was tiring. We had to stop the first at midnight, put on the cortisone and then start the second bag at 1 o'clock, not to mention the 4 o'clock check and the end of the chemo at 4:30 ... or vice versa. Before dad takes me home, the nurse calls someone for a reflexology session because she finds me tired.

I come home nauseous, with tinnitus, a great general malaise in my body and restless sleep. I'm totally out of touch, I don't really understand what is going on around me. I spend my time under my duvet or act as a robot for basic needs. I struggle with my body… I am in terrible pain.

A week after my hospitalization, mum drops me off at Christelle's for an energy treatment. After talking, she invites me to lie down on the massage table. While making circles on my stomach, she makes me inhale and exhale deeply. It's true that I don't take the time to breathe… I'm like snorkeling. Then she starts massaging my scalp, I apologize for the texture of my hair that the new chemos make «elastic». Christelle asks me to visualize a path, my path, on which there is a mountain of more or less heavy stones. These obstacles are for me to push or climb. She adds that my parents have their own paths, they can encourage me, but they will not be able to remove the stones for me. My tears are falling, but I don't know if it's painful or because the picture is beautiful. Then she massages my face with olive oil, it smells so good. Then the feet ... That I like less, I wince, but I really feel that it unlocks something in my back. With the only sound of relaxing music, Christelle washes her hands to massage my back, again with olive oil. So there ... This is the best. I totally relax, my body becomes light. After several minutes, which could have gone on for hours, she places a warm, wet towel on my back. At the end of the two hour session, she makes me draw an Oracle card from a pretty purple packet. I read «Life is beautiful» is a phrase that mum told me for a long time when I was pessimistic. Funny, because we just talked about parents. When I get home, I am thirsty and I ask mum to cook me some food. She points out to me that I went to Christelle's house, folded up on myself, but that I left with my shoulders back and straight. I can't believe how much help Christelle has been to me. It's a liberation.

I haven't been able to do anything for the past two weeks, but this morning I wanted to put on makeup! I haven't done it for a year! With my patches on my face and then exhaustion, I didn't see the point.

The home nurse takes my blood for the week and again it hurts. My veins are thin and I think my nurse doesn't like drawing blood too much. I report to the hospital that it is painful with every blood test and they advise me to change nurses at home. Before the stem cells are taken, my blood will have to be taken from my hands so that my veins at the folds of the elbows are preserved.

I help mum cook and she walks me to the fruit and veg store, but I'm the one driving! There's a crowd in the store, I'm looking for carrots, but everything looks like a carrot… or nothing. What does a carrot look like? It's blurry, I can't see anything. Phew! Mum arrives and takes back control of the shopping list. Illness never fails to remind me that I must rest.

Hard prick

"Do not lose hope,
you have to believe in it."

I'm in good shape and it's not hurting anywhere so it really bothers me having to go back to chemo tomorrow. I asked to go there on Monday to get out quickly. But as the afternoon draws to a close, the professor calls me to explain that they've had a lot of emergencies in the blood unit over the weekend and won't be able to accommodate me the next day. They will contact me tomorrow morning for an entry Tuesday or Wednesday. I am confused when my plans are changed at the last moment. I made a Reiki appointment with Christelle on Friday and want to be in good shape as soon as possible to go to the Tours fair which is Ireland themed.

Ireland is an important country to me, a country of heart. Since my first stay at the age of 17, my dream was to stay there for a few months. In 2016 I made that wish come true working in Cork for six months and stayed with a great big family, it was awesome. I am still in contact with them. My illness has affected them and they regularly hear from me. In fact, when I told my foster mom, Sheila, about my cancer, she worried about the hospital costs and about my comfort in the hospital. She was surprised to learn that I did not pay anything and that I was in a single room in a public hospital in good condition. I look forward to seeing them again as soon as I get better. In addition, with our parents, we plan to leave at the end of August in Scotland to mark the end of the treatments.

Monday morning, 11 a.m., rebound. The hospital calls me, casually, to tell me that my arrival is maintained today at 3 pm. I am shaking and nauseous. I quickly call dad to let him know, he's the one taking me and Loudun is an hour from Tours.

I put my things in my room, I do not forget my tablecloth to give it a little color. A caregiver I am seeing for the first time arrives in my room for inventory.

- Can we define my meals for the three days?
- It's the inventory or the dishes, I don't have time to do both.
- The dishes ! I have trouble eating in the hospital so this is most important.
- You won't have to complain about the inventory afterwards.

I don't leave my room, food is essential. I want as many comfort food as possible.

- Well! It's not all that balanced! Mash and pasta, she said sharply.

I laugh and add that on top of that, I'm constipated right now.

- If you are constipated, do not take a banana! she replies exasperated.

With the stress, I couldn't eat all day. Tonight, carbonara pasta is on the hospital menu. I ask timidly, to the same nurse, if I can have a second tray.

- Ah, but it had to be said if it was double serving every time! I have to write it down!

This nursing assistant is the exception, because in this service the medical team is very caring. The evening ends with the little happiness of having had some carbonara pasta.

On 30th April 2019, second day at the hospital, today it has been a year since I was first told about my cancer so today is Flavien's birthday. I have noticed that every year between March and May there is a wave of lymphoma diagnoses. Certainly, that little winter cold that begins to worry us with the onset of spring.

A day in the hospital is busy, here are 24 hours with me:

7:45 a.m. - Breakfast
8:20 a.m. - Taking of the constants by a nursing assistant
8:45 a.m. - Two times in my room, but I'm in the shower
8:55 a.m. - The caregiver collects breakfast
9:00 a.m. - The nurse gives me my medication
9:10 a.m. - The nurse adds a bandage so that my PAC remains airtight
10:20 a.m. - 30 minutes with the hypnotherapist
11:00 a.m. - Nap
11:15 a.m. - Room cleaning by two caregivers
12:00 p.m. Meal
12:30 p.m. - The announcing nurse comes to explain the autologous transplant to me
1:10 p.m. - Removal of the tray
1:20 p.m. - «A coffee? A tea ? «
1:21 p.m. - Art therapist
1:40 p.m. - External visit
1:50 p.m. - «You are going to the EFS in 10 minutes to have your veins checked,» the nurse warns me.
2:45 p.m. - Return to your room
3:30 p.m. - The announcement nurse returns
4:10 p.m. - Checking that the heart is functioning properly by electrodes
4:30 p.m. - Taking of constants by a caregiver
4:40 p.m. - 40 minutes with the hospital psychologist
6:00 p.m. - HAPPY BIRTHDAY, FLAVIEN! But I doze off

What about at night?

8:40 p.m. - Nurses pass by and I fall asleep
10:05 p.m. - End of chemo alarm
11:00 p.m. - Taking of constants
11:05 p.m. - Product rinsing
11:15 p.m. - Cortisone bag
11:20 p.m. - Return of blood to check the PAC
11:25 p.m. - Chemo launch
11:30 p.m. - Xanax to calm me down
11:50 p.m. - I'm cold, my cheeks are on fire, from cortisone and the smell of plastic in my pockets makes me nauseous
2:20 a.m. - End of chemo
03:25 - 10 minutes of rinsing
04:20 a.m. - Change of the hydration infusion and taking of the constants
8:15 am - Woken up by Pauline, my favorite nurse, and a new day at the hospital begins.

I am coming home after three days in the hospital, the effects are terrible, I feel like I am in a bubble with the tinnitus. I throw up a lot and the rest of the time I'm nauseous. Some days I lose my appetite and especially my taste, I have difficulty drinking. I am sick and my nightly awakenings do not help me. I have chills, I have a tachycardia, it hurts all over, I am weak, I have a nosebleed and I am leaking urine. It's bordering on bearable and if I lived next to a bridge I think I would have jumped. Nothing's going well and don't tell me that keeping my morale up is 50% off, it's the best way to make me feel guilty for being sad, upset, exhausted!

Mum comes to take care of me whenever she can. This midday, she's making nice slices of ham and cheese from Abondance for me. It smells good I want to devour them all. I swallow my first bite and straight away I feel bad. I see cloudy and dark, but I rush upstairs to my bed, shouting:

- AAAH I'm leaving! AAAH I'm leaving!

Mum follows me running. I don't know how I got to my bed. I feel this terrible discomfort again. Mum tries to calm me down by massaging my back. My body calms down. We analyze all the times I have had this sensation and the one thing in common is ... cheese! Wow.

- But I love cheese! The four-cheese pizza, the hot goat cheese ...

Nevertheless, I am ready to do anything not to feel bad like this again. So I will have to eat only pasteurized cheeses.

SOS Vol. 2
Playlist
LECTURE ALÉATOIRE
Tout oublier
Angèle et Roméo Elvis
À la vie à l'amour
Soprano
Le coach
Soprano
Donnez-moi
Les frangines
La grenade
Clara Luciani

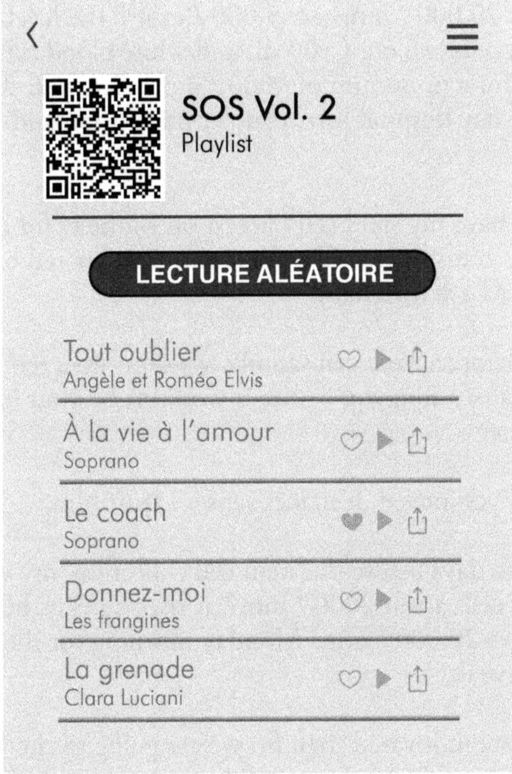

The time is long. Lying down, I watch the path of a spider on the ceiling. I can't go and dislodge her so high. She's more active than me. She does her life at her own pace. This one is rather beautiful in addition. As small as a pin-head, with well-proportioned little legs. I take the time to think about who is right between those who say the house is healthy if there are spiders and those who say it is poorly insulated. We definitely want to go to a house where we feel good, right?

Fifteen days after my treatments, I start to poke my head out of the water, I regain my strength. I have some bone pain that appears from Zarzio's bites, but it is a sign that my white blood cells are recovering. However, my blood test is catastrophic. Platelets which should not be below 20,000 / mm^3 are 5,000 / mm^3! The level of red blood cells is 8.6 g / 100 dL and white blood cells at 20 / mm^3 for a minimum of 4000 / mm^3. The next day, I go to the day hospital for a platelet transfusion and dad takes me.

- I have my stem cell harvest on Monday for my autologous transplant, will it do it with the few red blood cells I have? I ask internally.

- Before a stem cell sample, we don't do a red blood cell transfusion, you realize it wouldn't be your blood, she tells me.

Ah yes indeed, it makes sense. I trust him.

Two days before the stem cell collection, my white blood cells are at 2000 / mm^3, it rises quickly, but it is imperative 20,000 / mm^3 Monday morning for the sample. I believe it !

More motivated than fit, we are going to the Tours exhibition fair. My heart still beats quickly and I regularly have to sit in my folding seat which we now walk around everywhere. But I have no pain. We wandered around for almost two hours to see the exhibit, listen to live Irish music, and have a bite to eat. We come home, the weather is fine, we take advantage of our little garden. I take a nap and then I'm hungry for red meat so we're going to a restaurant to end the day well together.

I arrive at 9 am for the sample at the EFS (French Blood Establishment) accompanied by dad. The nurse takes my blood to check my white blood cell count and red blood cell count. The nurses have doubts that my red blood cell count was already low.

- Of course a prior transfusion is possible if necessary. There you are very weak. Red blood cells are not collected, they serve as a «mat» for optimal collection. The higher they are, the thicker the mat.

I try to stay calm, but I'm angry with this intern who pretended to know what she was talking about!

«What you know, knowing that you know;
what we don't know, to know that we don't know: is to really know.»
Confucius

It's not a shame not to know, you can't know everything. But when we are not in control, we are silent! We are going to find out, but we do not pretend to know everything, because MADAME is going to become a doctor. This is not the first to do this to me! It makes me angry every time.

We will still attempt the sample. At around 11 a.m., a catheter was placed in the crease of the right elbow. My blood is filtered in a centrifuge which retains more stem cells than usual in the blood by injecting them to stimulate production. Then my blood returns to where it came from, through the other arm. So I don't lose anything. As soon as I raise my arm too far, the machine will ring and vibrate to signal that the flow is not constant. I can't use my phone too much, luckily I was chatting with dad and watched a movie. In my right hand, I squeeze a bullet shaped like a drop of blood. I take this opportunity to spread the message on Instagram about the importance of donating blood.

After almost five hours of sampling, lying down without being able to move, the EFS team sent me to the blood unit to receive bags of blood. They doubt that the «harvest» of the stem cells was successful and programs me to take another sample the next morning. The wait is long, I am going to sleep in the hospital since my first bag will arrive around 11 pm. I'm going to have three pockets, a great first for me to have so many all at once. Checkups are frequent during a transfusion to make sure everything is going well so I don't get much sleep. But the night is nice, with the intern there are two students to whom he explains the whole procedure. It's super interesting and I'm participating as much as them! Even though I'm exhausted, I try to make this restless night a good time. The third and final bag of blood arrives at 7 a.m. and I return to the EFS at 9 a.m. Even though the building is next door, it is detached from the hospital, so we do the 500 meters ... by ambulance! It's the same nursing team today, that reassures me. They inform me that yesterday there were 3.59 / 4 collected, they did not expect such a good result. So they will reconnect me for less time today, but still three hours! The collection is done, the stem cells will be sent and frozen in Angers until I receive my last chemo, which will destroy all of my blood cells.

There is only a week to go before I go back to the hospital, and again I don't feel like it, because I'm in good shape! I've read that blueberries are good against tumor cells, so Flavien sets foot in our garden. I also take the opportunity to go shopping with mom. I can't stand my bras anymore, they compress me. I hope it is not the masses that are getting fat.

Monday 20th May, chemo day in weekly hospitalization and not in hematology. The doctor from the ward comes to see me. I see her often, she is sweet and smiling. She really takes my tinnitus into consideration and finds it surprising that it is not noted in the file when I pointed it out the last time ... internally! This is a fairly common effect to be taken seriously, as tinnitus can be irreversible ... so we switch to another product. I'm going from a 24 hour product with a six hour front check for my kidneys to a one hour product! This is completely crazy ! These are "cousin" products which have the same actions. But why didn't I have this treatment from the start? More expensive ? Less tested? We're confused with dad. This is a change that seems drastic. Will he act well? If that can limit all the other effects, that would be great. The previous two cycles were so difficult and painful.

I recognize the nurse who gives me the IV, her name is Amandine, I met her last year in this same department. She explains to me that she is there as a backup, but also to meet me, because she has changed jobs, she is now a nurse to support 16-25 year olds. It's new, it's great! I'm excited, that's great news. Amandine will come back tomorrow and take the time to tell me about her role.

Regularly, during my hospitalizations, a socio-esthetician comes to offer me a treatment. I always choose the hands because protecting your nails is important, but I don't always have the strength to apply a base and two coats of polish. It's a nice moment, she massages my hands for a long time with moisturizer before applying the polish. It motivates me to go for treatment.

The first bag is placed at 5 pm then the product from 3 am to 6 pm. Right now I have no side effects, I just wait 11:30 p.m. for someone to come and take the chemo pump off. I constantly get up to urinate. It's 3 am, I'm not sleeping, I'm upset, so I'm writing about my relationship to food. Nothing crazy, but maybe it will be a future post for my blog. Since 2007, I have been writing on the internet. I'm mainly talking about creative hobbies, a few travelogues to remember it, and recently some articles on the disease, but I certainly don't want that to be the dominant theme. Initially, I wrote little and progressed over the years, especially thanks to my end-of-studies internship where I wrote articles for a web magazine about Touraine. It has become a passion!

The day goes by, as do the people in my room. No time to doze off; chemo installation at 8:15 am, visit of the youth nurse, dietitian, art therapist, my referring doctor, the ward doctor... Since I am staying only one night in the hospital, at 3 pm I can already run away! I feel like I'm less in pain than last time around, I really hope the effects weren't so bad. I'll see tomorrow. Will this chemo rhyme with insomnia? I had so much cortisone. I am walking on eggshells with this situation, expecting myself to feel terrible at any time.

After a week, I already manage to do several things, this chemo is much more livable! I didn't have a suicidal desire. Sure, I'm exhausted and nauseous, but less and the appetite is back. The tinnitus has subsided, I can watch TV even though the noise of the vacuum cleaner and plastic bags still annoys me.

It's the last long weekend in May, we're going to our parents's house. Flavien goes kayaking on the Vienne for a day and I take advantage of my grandparents who come to eat in Loudun. But my blood test this morning is bad and the hospital call is not long in coming to schedule a blood and platelet transfusion tomorrow. Mum takes me to the hospital, Flavien stays in Loudun to celebrate his brother's 30th birthday. I am upset to miss the evening and not be able to see Blandine's round belly pregnant with their second child expected in August. The only positive note of the day, I will be able to rest and be «in shape» for Monday's PET scan.

- Your PET scan is not as good as we expected. There are still masses left, my doctor tells me the day after my exam.

My body doesn't want me anymore!

It is not possible !

Was I tortured by chemo for nothing ?!

The autologous transplant is therefore postponed and in the meantime I will have different chemotherapy drugs. I had gotten used to the idea of going on an autologous transplant in June. Another change of plan.

I'm afraid of dying. It is a delicate subject to discuss with those close to me. It's simple, they refuse to talk about it. I don't want my life to be shortened because of cancer. I am too curious to see how my life and that of others will evolve. I am curious to go and explore as many countries as possible. I have new things to learn. It would hurt my parents too much. Just kidding, I repeat to them that they should have had at least one more child, maybe this one wouldn't have been missed. And Flavien has invested so much ... he will have wasted a lot of time with me. And I want to continue to live lots of beautiful moments with him. The phrase grandpa utters every Christmas is spinning in my head. «I might not be here next year.» What if it's me? Who would come to my funeral? Not many people! For there to be a minimum number of people, it must absolutely be a Saturday ... Or a public holiday! Are funerals done on a public holiday? I was never afraid to die. At least not until I realized my dream of moving to Ireland. I see myself on the plane home, after seven months in this country, thinking:

- What if I died in this plane crash?

From that moment on, I was not only afraid of MY death, but also of MY death. In my phone, I start an instruction note if I die. My passwords, the song I wish for my funeral… I don't want a coffin, I have discovered urns where the body is used as fertilizer for a tree. Since I cannot donate my organs, as much as I use to nourish a tree. If I am a fruit tree, an apricot tree, my fruit will look small and sweet, but in reality it will be sour to say, «Don't bother! It fits my temper well. I entrust my anxieties to the psychologist at the hospital before my doctor explains to me the care that will be put in place.

- Do not be afraid to suffer, there are palliative chemotherapy drugs.

In addition, she offers me a document to register my last wishes, advance directives. I am learning that I can easily find it on the internet. I just wanted to be reassured, to hear that all is not lost. But listening to him, we have to believe that he is. I came out devastated. It was as if she had validated all of my concerns.

A clock without a needle

Time stands still. Everything must be day to day. Impossible to foresee anything for more than a fortnight. In fact, my hematologist forbade me to plan, so I wouldn't be disappointed to cancel. It is best to organize at the last moment and with cancellation insurance. It's frustrating, I need deadlines to move forward. I like to have goals, projects that motivate me every day and make my days too short. Without all of that, life seems bland to me. I who was always in the preparation of future trips and the organization, everything must have a plan B and often plan B is the cancellation. I can't wait for the disease to disappear, it is becoming much too long. I see my friends going on vacation, setting up their business, buying a house, having a baby ... All of this is impossible for me, I feel stuck there. It's life in the conditional, for example, if I'm fine we'll go to La Rochelle.

I'm in better shape, I take the opportunity to do creative hobbies, it makes me feel good. A birthday card for grandma, linocut and a macrame feather. I also accepted a video interview for a local magazine, we are going to talk about my blog and social media. This is my first time doing a filmed interview, I'm afraid to sound silly, but I'm surprised how quickly I feel comfortable with the crew.

Flavien agrees to accompany me to the psychologist I met during the focus group at IETO37. She receives many families and couples in her office. It will do him good to be able to talk to someone outside. I feel guilty for causing him to suffer the disease and I am proud that he has the shoulders to take it all and that he hasn't run away.

Return of treatment
Live better the side effects
Buy popsicles
Make my toothpaste
coconut oil to remove bandage glue

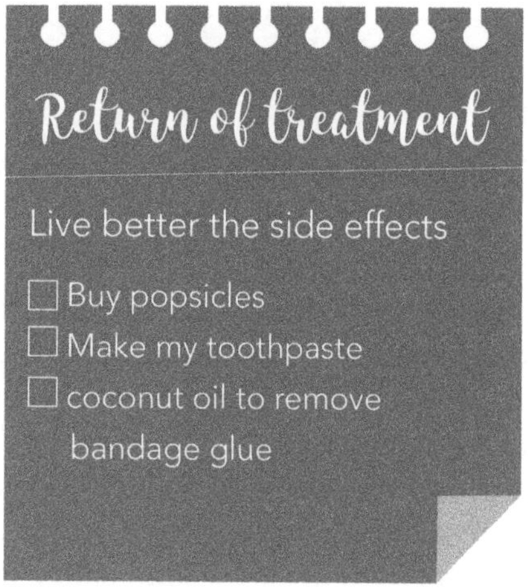

Thursday 13th June, I have a new two-day chemo protocol coupled with antibodies, the same ones I will have in treatment after the autologous transplant. At 4 p.m. the psychologist from the hospital comes for a final explanation with me. The last one, because I don't want to see her again.

- When I tell you throughout the conversation that I'm afraid of dying and you don't answer me ...
- I answered, you didn't hear.
- So what did you say?

She is silent before resuming.

- I'm not here to give you medical answers or to comfort you. You were waiting for medical answers.
- I was wondering about the other treatments available! What should I talk to you about if I can't share my

concerns? Of my radishes that grow in my garden? I collected four, I am delighted! If it's like that, I'd rather call my grandma!

She laughs… Not me!

- If you change your mind, I won't blame you and will come back for psychological support.

Except it's on me to blame him! It's over !

The new chemo is bearable, although three days after leaving hospital I am very ill. It makes me late for my ENT appointment. The hearing test reveals a slight loss of hearing in the treble. My tinnitus is less intense, the doctor explains to me that it should decrease and depend on my fatigue. I'm moving to the day hospital for my thirteenth and fourteenth red blood cell transfusions.

- Thank you donor number thirteen, I say sincerely looking at the blood bag.

The young nurse laughs next to me. I don't know if donors realize how much relief they give people. From this first pocket, I will feel less breathless and my pale complexion will turn pink.

This year, I'm enjoying the music festival, in a small town near Tours. With Flavien, we join his colleague Simon. I've only seen him twice, but he's the kind of person who gets the hang of it right away. He is comfortable with the illness and always gently asks how I am and I am confident to tease him like an old friend. Flavien's friends live mainly in the south of France, I don't know them much since I fell ill at the start of our relationship. He regularly has to refuse weekends and cannot accommodate them at home. It's difficult in terms of social ties. Little by little, the emptiness is created around us. Isolation due to our out of step life. Fortunately, in addition to my parents, I have my in-laws. They are always present and very attentive. I am comfortable with them and I do not hesitate to talk to them about everything.

The end of June is rather calm, it is hot in Tours, luckily we have reserved a weekend in La Rochelle where it is twenty degrees cooler! We even have to buy sweaters. We walk a lot to explore the city. We walk so much that on the last day I was on the verge of collapsing on our walk on the beach. The sand is a thousand needles under my feet, it's unbearable. My legs don't carry me anymore, Flavien has to hold me. Quick, quick that I sit down in the car and we go back to Tours.

Hard prick

“ ... Hold on my dear.
Did they give you an end of life date? ”

A few days later, before going to meet a naturopath ... I eat a burger. I understand the benefits of «healthy» food on the body, but I am not ready to sacrifice so much. Especially on days when eating is my only pleasure. I like to discover restaurants, I have a long list of restaurants to try in Tours. Two things make me happy: food and creative hobbies.

Thursday 4th July, chemo day. Yesterday, the hospital called to tell me to come at 10 am instead of 3 pm and finally my chemo arrived at 5 pm, just after Elodie, the art therapist. We had an interesting conversation about the present moment and the philosophy of life in India, which she goes to regularly. For them, only the present moment exists. There is no past or future, that's their secret to happiness. Do not wait to be well to live. Time is no longer an inexhaustible resource when you are sick. «I will do it next year or in five years,» those words are no longer thoughtlessly said.

Except right now I'm nauseous! The fresh pineapple juice helps me a bit. In the days following chemo, I mainly eat fruit. Good, sweet and juicy peaches. It's the only food that tempts me, but my stomach doesn't seem to like it as much as I do.

Since May, Laurine has been coming to do my blood tests. The first few times I thought she was talking very loudly, but now I realize that with the fatigue I was in slow motion and all the sounds were amplified. I like this nurse very much, we are almost the same age, she is bubbly, she takes the time to chat and she never hurts me. I did well to dare to change it. The day's blood work shows another drop in red blood cells, but the transfusion can wait. Fortunately, because we are leaving for three days in Brittany, towards Saint-Malo. The pretty Emerald Coast amazes us. Flavien and I have a crush on this region. We are once again making great restaurants and I am eating my first mussels. I tasted the Flavien dish in La Rochelle and liked it so this time I chose a large plate just for myself. The weather is nice, not too hot. We stay in Airbnb, with a French-Scottish couple. We take the time to chat with them over breakfast. How nice to hear English spoken. Fatigue blocks me and can't speak a single word of English. I, who adore this language, am disappointed. But it was a great meeting!

In the evening, it is astonishment when I learn that Jennifer has died of b lymphoma. It's so cruel. She was born only three days after me, in 1994. She had a very difficult treatment journey, the autologous transplant had not worked and she recently received a new American treatment called CarT cells. Yet it was a promising treatment. I find it hard to understand how this is possible. I also feel fear, it makes death even more present.

Monday 22nd July, the end of our stay in Brittany is strange, sadness mixed with the desire to take full advantage of the moment. We're heading back to Tours just in time to pick up my EPO bite from the pharmacy for tomorrow. I need them, the lack of red blood cells makes me breathless with the slightest effort.

Three days later, I arrive at the hospital and tell about my trip to Saint-Malo, I explain that now I like mussels. But the nurse tells me that it is strongly discouraged, even if it is cooked it remains a seafood. room laughing.

- Well then, we eat mussels? This is not good!

I quickly get disillusioned, my white blood cells are too low so the chemo won't start today or tomorrow. Obviously when we change my plans… I cry! It is 40 ° C outside and 27 ° C at home, the healthcare team suggests that I sleep in the hospital tonight and come back after the weekend. Amandine, the youth nurse, helps me find the positive of the situation: Tuesday, I will be able to meet two young people at the art therapy workshop.

In addition, the lag in my chemo allows me to go to my grandparents where my cousin, who now lives in Toulouse, comes to eat with his girlfriend. We meet Élisa and Valentin finally meets Flavien. We usually only see each other at Christmas, it feels good to spend the afternoon with them. The conversation often turns into debate with our different opinions and characters, but he is a caring cousin.

So on Tuesday 30th July, I'm going back to the hospital for the third round of chemo with the antibodies. This afternoon, I am going to the art therapy workshop. I'm so impatient, it's 2pm and I'm ready when it's only half an hour away. This is the first time that I have met young people in the hospital. I'm early, Élodie, the art therapist is already here, she is preparing the workshop in the large bright room which overlooks the entrance to the hospital and a park. Léo also arrives, at only 17 he has osteosarcoma, and he will receive his very first chemo tonight. He looks relaxed. His long blonde hair immediately reminds me of all the inches he could give Solid'Hair, I have to tell him about it! Léo is preparing an artistic baccalaureate, he does not waste time to start creating. As for me, I am undertaking the making of a butterfly origami. At 3 pm, I quickly return to my room to have the nurse give me my hour-long chemo. At 4 p.m., after just one butterfly, because I was mostly talking, I have to go to the ward to turn off the chemo pump. Speaking has whetted my appetite, I ask the caregiver for a cupcake. Leaving my room, I greet a granny who is in the hallway. The old lady follows me down the halls leading to the art therapy room, maybe she wants to steal my cake? She is a regular at the workshop, she settles around the table. Then comes, timidly, Angeline. At 19, she has been in chemo for nine months for osteosarcoma as well.

- Above all, we must remain positive, confides the grandmother.
- A friend told me «We undergo the negative, we create the positive», I add.

She loves it and wants someone to write it down for her on a piece of paper. Élodie grabs a nice piece of paper, Léo draws a flower and Angeline punches a dragonfly in her watercolor. It forms an egregore of positive energies that do us all good. At 5:30 p.m. the workshop has to stop, I only made two origami butterflies, but got to talk about the hair donation, Léo seemed excited about the idea.

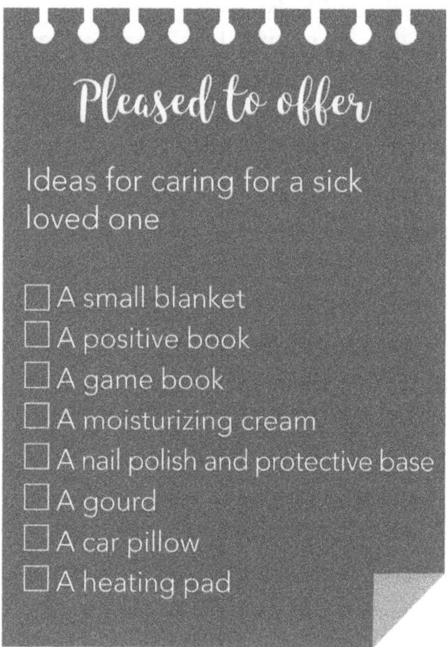

I'm fed up with being locked up since being released from the hospital, on that first day of August, I decide it's time to have my hair shaved. Flavien comes with me to Line's salon Artist in Herbs. We cry almost as much as we joke. The next day, Flavien suggests that his parents go for a drink at the Rochecorbon tavern. It's hot, the turban is not comfortable, I take it off confidently just 30 minutes after our arrival. It is especially the elderly who wonder. Some do not take their eyes off me. A few people have the gentle gaze of compassion and I see the gaze of those who have gone through this ordeal. They are often accompanied by a small sigh. These looks are heartwarming.

The nausea does not leave me, the treatments weigh on me. It's heavy ! I can't wait to get well. Christelle soothes me during my Reiki session, she explains to me that I am a caterpillar in her cocoon. I'm preparing to be a butterfly, but I need some time before I spread my wings. It is a beautiful picture of the disease.

The lack of red blood cells means Flavien can hear my heart beating. Obviously, a few days later, mum and dad have to take me to my 15th and 16th blood transfusion. My blogger friend, Camille, takes the opportunity to come see me after her plasma donation. I'm glad she's taking the time to chat with me. It is thanks to her book and her blog «Camille is launching» that I pay more attention to ecology. At 3 p.m., it's over, I say a quick hello to Angeline, who is in chemo in an upstairs room, before going back to rest.

The days go by and I am getting closer to my entry into autograft. I'm waiting for the call from the hospital to know the result of my PET scan. We take the opportunity to visit a few surrounding towns and see friends almost every day and even friends that I had not seen for 10 years. Indeed, while some have avoided me, others have kindly come back for news. This helps put grudges aside.

Despite these beautiful times, I am stressed and I'm in low spirits, so tonight, on a whim, Flavien told me:

- Let's go bowling!

I think of a joke, I smile, but no, we are actually going bowling together. We have a great time, we have mocktails and we have a lot of fun. Of course, I lose, but very few points! It was really a great idea.

The next day, I decide to call the hospital to find out about the result.

- It's off to a good start, this chemo worked, but there are still a few masses left. For me, it will be good for the autograft, but we have to wait for the multidisciplinary decision, my doctor tells me.

Thursday 15th August, we celebrate Lucas' three years. He has to go around the table to give thank-you kisses, but it's my turn ...

- Not Laura! Not Laura! he cries out as my tears start to fall.

I don't have my turban, maybe that's it. But I'm wearing makeup, with colorful earrings that's more of a style. He heard that I was sick so he's scared? When you are little, you can catch a disease. "Don't go out without a coat, you'll be sick". I do not know.

The week preceding my entry into autograft, we have a restaurant almost every day. I absolutely want to give Flavien a taste of poutine. This Quebec specialty that I adored during my stay in Quebec a few years ago. Unfortunately, there are none in Tours, so we go to Châtellerault where our parents meet us. We are also testing the Coffee Shop that a childhood friend opened in Saumur.

I absolutely wanted to see Nicole and her daughter Maëlle whom I consider to be my cousin. So I invite them to Tours. We do what we love to do together, we have a snack! Nicole gives me a stone bracelet, which has the virtue of stimulating the immune system. Very symbolic, I will take him with me for an autograft.

Thursday 22th August, 2019 is the big day. I walk into the hospital at 3:30 p.m. I forgot the patch to put on my PAC again. I quickly hooked up, but I have to wait for the doctor to come by to explain everything to me before launching the product. At 6 p.m. Flavien arrives at the hospital, he left work early. Three quarters of an hour later, the doctor comes into my room and explains to me that they are reluctant to go on a double autograft, two autografts four months apart.

- Okay, but in the meantime I start anyway?
- No, there will be no chemo today or tomorrow. You will be back on Monday while we make a decision with the department professor and the other doctors.
- I do not understand why.
- They are not the same products.
- What makes you hesitate?
- The PET scan shows a response of over 90%, which is good, but not perfect. If it is a single it will be the BEAM protocol and if it is a double BAM.

The names of the protocols at least offer the advantage of making us laugh, but I'm completely confused, it had to be the big day and eventually it will be from Monday. I struggle with this kind of change which is usual in the hospital. The team is rushing to get me unplugged and leave quickly. To change our minds, with my parents and Flavien, we go to a restaurant, but that doesn't stop me from crying. I had everything planned, I was organized, prepared. Coming in today made me have mom's help longer before she went back to work. Even at 25 having a mum is reassuring.

I keep my head busy until Monday, watch playoffs and make bracelets for everyone. I try to choose the colors for each one. This is my way of showing my presence in case this goes wrong. It's not easy to take your mind off things, I think about the fact that I should be on chemo, and since I am not, tonight is pizza!

I can even be present during the cousinade in Flavien's family. More than fifty people! Last year I was too weak to kiss everyone, I could barely stand. And this year, no kisses either, I must not catch any virus so as not to be sick during the autologous transplant. I pass for an alien to repeat «Hello from afar».

Monday 26th August, day of anguish because I am expected at 3 pm at the hospital for the autologous or double autologous transplant. At the end of the afternoon, the doctor arrives and announces the double autograft and the start of chemo tomorrow morning. The first three days, I will have a two hour chemo bag every six hours. My dreaded caregiver, the one who criticized my meal choices in April, walks into my room. Strangely, she is very nice, she comes to give me advice on autologous transplantation. I am suspicious and let mum do the talking.

- Don't you have your fluff with you today? she asks me.

Since the last time I saw her, I have shaved my hair and so… she is mistaking me for someone else! I laugh inside. Are all bald people the same?

August 27th 2019, two rooms, two atmospheres.
10 am, Tours hospital, start of the first major chemo for my autograft.
10 am, Chinon hospital, birth of Flavien's second nephew, Léandre.

It's a shame that there isn't an art therapy workshop, because I'm in good shape, I have few side effects. I take advantage of the embroidery to occupy my hands and mind, because in a sterile room it will not be allowed. The instructions are strict there, my clothes must be washed at sixty degrees then put in the dryer and put, separately, in freezer bags. Anything that cannot be washed cannot enter the room.

Mum takes me some frozen meals, a variety of pasta dishes that the hospital allows me to store in their fridge.

I can no longer see their dull speckled beige platters. And the towels disgust me ... The same ones I had as a child in the canteen, red or green, checkered. Just thinking about it makes me gag.

My second night was lulled by the comings and goings of the medical team. I fell asleep at 9 p.m., but at 11 p.m. the third bag of chemo arrived. At 1 a.m. the rinse was started, then the machine stopped at 2 a.m. At 3 a.m., one of the three pumps began to chime. A shrill beep because she was out of battery. I am implementing a strategy so that the machines are fully charged so that I don't wake up and have to unplug them in the middle of the night to go to the bathroom.

It's 5 a.m., the time for the fourth bag of chemo, followed by 7 a.m. for the rinse. At 7:30 am, the nurse takes my constants and at 8:00 am she offers me breakfast, which I refuse. I have my routine, in the morning I'm going to have my cappuccino and a croissant with mum and dad in the cafeteria. Flavien is working, but he doesn't forget to send me a message when he gets up.

At the start of the afternoon with mum and dad, we join Angeline and her mum to chat. At the end of the hall, there is a table and chairs, the place is bright with large windows, it changes the rooms. There is a library with some pretty old books and a few games, nothing interesting. The hypnotherapist offers us both a session while our parents continue to discuss. Even though we are no longer children, it is a difficult context for them and talking to other parents who are going through the same situation is essential. The hospital offers «caregivers' coffee», this meeting takes place once a month, but in the middle of the week so mum has never been able to make it.

Hard prick

> “We do not ask you for news because we see that you are not dejected.”

The days go by and I lose track of time. My memories are fuzzy, I don't remember who happened or when. I am not in pain, I am not nauseous, but the fatigue is overwhelming.

Last morning before entering the sterile room. The cappuccino is difficult to pass and I leave half of the croissant. Something is changing. I go back to my room and after a few minutes I throw up my super breakfast. I am completely exhausted and collapse to the floor, with the door still open. The nurses come running for fear that I might pass out.

There you have it, that really sounds like the end of freedoms for several weeks.

Now is the time to switch off your brain. Everyone is proceeding as they see fit for this difficult stage. For my part, I am going to a desert island, no one, nothing to think about. I have had too many testimonials from girls who were caged lions in their small, sterile rooms. If I set a day out for myself, it's going to be a blast.

I observe myself, I observe the situation from the outside. My head is totally dissociated from my body. I am not allowed to have my notebook, it is mum who will note my feelings for the next few days.

It starts with ...

A shower, with a specific product and a clean outfit that the hospital lends me. Then I go into the sterile room. It's not unknown to me since it's where I slept the very first time I came to the hematology department. I hope this will be the last room I spend so much time in.

I panic. The ward nurse sees him and comes to my height next to my bed. She grabs my hand and asks which shows I like. Talking to him instantly calms me down. She had the right reflex, that's lovely of her.

It's my doctor's turn to enter the room, along with her intern.

- I'm on vacation for the rest of your hospitalization, she announces, it's Raphaël, my intern, who will take over.

Following the setbacks I have had with internal precedents, I wonder. But these days, this intern has shown his seriousness, I just have to trust him completely. He is now my only point of reference.

At the end of the afternoon, the caregiver comes into my room and pulling on the pants that I am wearing, she exclaims:

- It's okay, we don't bother! These are our pants!

I have no vouch for this kind of person. I have only one fear now, staring at that door ... whether it be her. I hear the first airlock door open, but I can't see who is in the decompression airlock. Before entering my sterile room, everyone should put on a charlotte, gown, overshoes and mask. Only three people are allowed in the room, myself included.

On September 3, the team gathered around me to put a gastric tube on me, but the pocket of stem cells arrived at the same time. The gastric tube is difficult to pass, it irritates my whole throat. Even when drinking at the same time through a straw to aid insertion, it is an extremely unpleasant sensation, especially when passing through the throat. A second nurse comes in to infuse my arm, it's better for the stem cells. Everything takes place in absolute calm. At least in my head. I am at ease, because I know that I am in good hands and supported by the hypnotherapist. Unable to infuse my arms or hands and time is running out, the stem cells have to «go home» quickly after they take them out of the freezer. Eventually, the medical team decides to send them through the PAC.

Mum walks into my room, she passed the nurses who told her that it had not gone as planned. The lead paused longer than expected and the radiologist was unable to verify that the lead was properly placed to remove the wire that guides the insertion. Time was ticking and the graft was at its thaw limit, a few more minutes and it was out of use. I haven't achieved any of this.

The night shift puts down the feeding bag, the hose also goes through a pump to prevent air bubbles. The feeling of liquid, cold food that goes down my throat and settles in my stomach is… unique! And sickening! I gag and feel uncomfortable all the time. And in the night, what had to happen, happened. I vomit. Part of the catheter comes out through my nose and the other through my mouth. What to do ? Reinsert it? I do not want it anymore ! In the middle of the night, I ring the crying medical staff. The night nurse reassures me:

- There are other solutions besides the probe which is really not easy to bear.

Indeed, the next day the intern informed me that I will be fed by the PAC. It will provide nutrients to my blood, but will not work my stomach. So I will only have kept the probe for twelve hours. Dirty probe! I wish I had let myself be convinced. Now I can't swallow my saliva, I have to spit it out in a tiny cardboard bowl called a «bean». Maybe if it weren't for the sore throat I would have eaten some crème caramel.

Fatigue, vomiting, diarrhea, mucositis... these could be the basic symptoms of a severe gastroenteritis. It's much more terrible than that. The body is exhausted. I don't eat or drink anything because I can't.

My days are punctuated by the medical team. I have no choice, I am entirely dependent on the nursing staff. While they disinfect my room, I wash at the sink, with a disposable glove. There is no shower in the bedroom and I am not allowed to use my toothbrush, instead I have a big cotton swab and mouthwashes. Twice a week, a physiotherapist makes me do exercises to prevent my muscles from melting too quickly. If I am too tired, I stay lying down and he adapts the exercises. A different extern comes every day since I entered the sterile room to give me a laser session in my mouth and reduce the mucositis which is invasive and painful. It didn't help my throat, it still hurts a lot when I swallow my saliva. Today, I'm dozing, I don't want to! I feel a breath, it's strange ... my eyes widen.

- But your mask! I tell her, completely hallucinated.

He sheepishly returns to the airlock to equip himself properly. I don't mind him forgetting the charlotte or the overshoes, but not the mask! Especially when he has to give me a treatment thirty centimeters from the face.

The beige food pouch arrives at 8 p.m. daily. I don't have the strength to look at the composition. And every day, an hour later, I vomit in pain, because I have nothing to throw up, my stomach is completely empty. I ask the night shift for beans and a nurse suggests that I go to the bathroom when I run out. But I need to be seated so much it pulls and constricts my stomach. She hands me new beans and leaves without worrying. It is so much of a habit for them in this department that they do not take the time to comfort me, to take my mind off me, which could have helped me.

Air conditioning blows continuously directly above my bed. Besides making a draft and a deafening noise, the smell of food or cigarettes invades my room several times a day.

- The air is taken from the outside, next to a door through which the meals enter for the service. This is also the place where some take a cigarette break even though we have already explained the problem to them, a nurse informs me.

They don't realize that in a sterile room you throw up nothing and besides, I'm a non-smoker! The air conditioning makes me cold at night, I'm only allowed a light sheet, and my sweatshirt doesn't keep me warm enough. To escape the breath on my head, I put on my hood, but it makes my head heat up and causes me to have a fever. And ... I'm still so cold! Who says fever at night, says blood culture sampling! To make sure I don't have an infection. While we are in the middle of the night and I want to sleep, the blood is drawn from both arms and not from the PAC, which takes a lot longer because a vein has to be found. And this blood sample is taken two or three consecutive nights.

At night the loneliness and fear are present, everything is more difficult, but I am adjusting as best I can by dealing with the problems one by one. In order to prevent my urine from overflowing the bin on the toilet, I empty it a little. However, I have to remember how many milliliters I pour out to tell the caregiver when she passes. This way, they make sure that my kidneys are working well between the products I get and what goes to the bathroom. I often urinate with all of these products.

The next day, with the caregiver, we establish a strategy. I take off my hood before taking the temperature, we also notice that my ear «warms» less. It works and makes us laugh every time.

My stool needs to be analyzed. After three exhausting tries during the day, I managed to do it in the small pot! I call and it's ... THE famous nurse's aide.

- Is that so ? Oh, but I don't know. I am going to ask.

Obviously, she does not come back and it is time for a change of team. I ring again, the night nurse has not been informed, the information has not been transmitted. She takes care of it immediately. The afternoon nurse's aide just didn't want to do it!

Hard prick

> " I feel lucky to win this straightener and I invite @lauranaudin to participate in this giveaway. "

This morning, it's Sarah, the caregiver I've known since the start of the treatments, who comes to clean the room. It makes me happy to see her, but impossible to discuss, I suffer terribly from hunger. I am writhing in pain. I cannot feed myself, my whole esophagus burns me, I ask for a Gaviscon, to try to appease like in the advertisement with the firefighters and the fire hose. I take my Gaviscon in pain, sip by sip. It relieves me a bit.

In view of the pain, I accept the increase in morphine. But from that moment on, I lose all my mental faculties. I doze, nightmare and hallucinate. I spend my whole night, even awake, in The Hunger Games. Obviously, in the morning the medical team laughs a lot and the information spreads quickly. Raphaël, the intern, comes in and asks me:

- Was that the Hunger Games? «Has fate been favorable to you?» «

I don't do it again on a night like this! Take it all off! I enjoyed watching the movies, but spending my night trying to be the sole survivor of the arena ... very little for me! Raphaël accepts that the morphine is reduced, but he warns me that the pain can come back. I have to make a choice between physical or psychological harm. Losing control of your head is unbearable so I confirm my choice to cut back on morphine.

The days go by ... I can't watch TV, but I want to follow Plus belle la vie on my phone, in rerun. If I'm not asleep, I kill myself with my phone, mindless scrolling, so I don't think about what I'm going through. When I'm awake, I accept visits, Flavien, Dad, Mum, or sometimes all three during the day if I'm really «fine». Usually very talkative, I don't always have the strength to talk to them.

During his daily visit, Raphaël takes the time to chat. This is my only medical connection, it comes several times a day. I have a huge chance to run into him after all these months with interns to watch out for. The interns work long hours, they stay late to write the day's reports. The medical team, meanwhile, changes almost every day, aisle, hour, shift ... It's rarely the same three days in a row.

- Above all, keep your humanity, I repeat.

But he always answers me:

- This is the first thing I lose!

He explains his school career to me, later I think about it and I realize by calculating his years of study that he is a year younger than me! It's strange that he's younger than me.

Every night I write a mini recap of my day to post on Instagram. A tiny part of the daily pain that I share to give news, keep track, and inform the Kopines who will pass by there.

In the morning, I wonder if the day will be better than the previous one. This morning, unexpectedly, the nurse and Raphael poke their heads through the door. A big smile and they chuckle.

- Guess what ?!
- White blood cells ?! I ask, my eyes widening.
- Yes ! They are at 1,200! Doors openning !

And they push open the door without having to put on the full outfit to enter my room. Too good, I'm going to discover the smiles hiding behind the masks and get out of the room a bit. I have permission to eat slowly. The body knows how to make itself understood. I have an inexplicable craving for milk! I would like to drink the bottle of milk! I swallow a few spoonfuls of the creme caramel, it goes well even though I hadn't eaten yogurt in years. I drink water again, a few sips. I am not yet ready for a full meal. But at dinner time ...

- A tray ? lovable saint asks me.
- No thank you, I have my creme caramel.

- Oh come on! It's carbonara tonight!
- No thanks.
- You like carbonara pasta, half!

This is one of my favorite dishes, so I accept and sit down at the table.

- Ah! It is true that you are boring you, you must not put the tray in the room, she adds.

Except that my gluttony will ruin me, after two bites I don't even have time to get up and throw everything up. I ring, she comes back to clean up, grumbling. I feel uncomfortable and make myself very small in my bed. The nurse and Raphael arrive. They reassure me:

- You can't eat hot, let alone something rich with cream. We told him not to force you to eat a meal.

It is true that I am terribly hungry, but between the pain to swallow and the rejection from my stomach, it's totally blocked. I note in my phone all the dishes that tempt me for my return home. My stomach is growling.

And the next day :

- So ? Aren't we throwing up tonight?

We will have recognized her ... she is the unfriendly caregiver!

The increase in white blood cells does not mean the end of the galleys. I am always hooked up to a multitude of products and I still vomit as much. Since the products no longer knock me out, I have insomnia. But my throat is getting better and better.

Wednesday September 18, after 24 days of hospitalization, Raphaël informs me that I can be discharged today, just after one last platelet transfusion. I thank him for his seriousness and his humanity. The art therapist and the hypnotherapist have been made aware and wish me a safe journey home.

- Oh no, but you're not going out today! the nurse, always the same, arrives in my room.
- Yes, I will wait for my platelets and then I go, I answer confidently.
- Ahah no, it's too late for the pads, it won't be before tomorrow!

No matter what, at 4 pm my platelets arrive as expected and the transfusion is quick. In two weeks, I had eight platelet transfusions.

I come out of my sterile room, mum is accompanying me with my luggage. I want to say goodbye to the great hemato team, but the ward is empty. The only one who appears at the end of the hall ... the nurse's aide ... Big hypocritical smile waving her arm in my direction.

It's not the ideal start, but at least I'm going home!

The eye of the needle
In French it's sound like the «cat» of the needle

It's nice to be in bed again. It's also strange, after a month of being watched I'm on my own. My toilet seems abnormal to me, the «pot» for separating urine is no longer present and the bowl is warm and comfortable. I feel like I am in another universe. And the noise, finally… the non-noise! The purr of the air conditioning didn't rock me at all. I don't have to carry around the IV stand I was attached to anymore. I had finally got used to it all, I was in a reassuring cocoon. My benchmarks are upset. If something happens, I don't have medical help.

When I got home from the hospital, a package was waiting for me. Lots of little touches that my 5th grade teacher sent me. Sixteen years later, illness brought us back in touch. Her heating pad is welcomed, I'm so cold.

Getting home is complicated. I did not expect this. Awakenings are frequent, to the rhythm of ghost visits by nurses. My duvet is so heavy, it pushes me against the mattress. I don't have the strength to move it so I switch to Flavien's duvet who is sleeping on the couch so I can rest. My rabbit night light, like the little ones, has never been so useful at night. When I wake up many times, she reminds me that I am indeed at home, in my bed. What a relief as soon as I see her!

It's really hard, my stomach and head are hungry, but I throw up what little I eat. It makes me despair. I don't know which organ in my body refuses this food. Yet Flavien's homemade mash tempted me so much. I only swallow a few tablespoons of the creme caramel. Food anguishes me and at the same time it obsesses me. I spend hours looking at recipes to keep me hungry. I don't know what to try to finally eat. My stomach twists with hunger in the night, so I take a tiny piece of madeleine that I barely swallow with a little water. I constantly have an iron taste in my mouth. In the hospital, I took sips of Pepsi on the recommendation of the medical team. It eases my nausea, but the bad taste persists so Nicole advises me to add a little sugar to my glass of water ... Miracle! My mouth is getting softer every day.

The five kilograms of water accumulated during the autologous transplant are drained and by eating so little I lose weight. I am at least three kilograms from my base weight. It's not huge, I'm not alarmed, but the dietician at the hospital is threatening to give me a gastric tube. For her, it's not normal to eat so little after being released from the hospital for three weeks. I categorically decline the probe, but she insists for forty-five minutes on the phone. I'm exhausted and wonder if she noticed that I ended the conversation in tears. The Kopines who have gone through autologous transplantation before me are unanimous in saying that the appetite is slowly returning. Coralie allays my concerns, it was the same for her when she left the hospital, it took her several weeks. On his advice, I drown some pasta under a natural yogurt and it goes. At my parents' house, mum prepares me platters with lots of things to make me want. Tonight, it's gruyère gougères. It's soft, it goes well, I'm doing it slowly, the aperitif tiles also work. I don't have too much taste anymore so I'm looking for crispness. I am upset, because I want to eat, everything tempts me, but impossible to swallow everything. On the morning tray, a peach, the last of the season, cereals softened with milk, a crème caramel, the safe bet, and water to swallow my two large medicines. But despite this help, I can't go a morning without throwing up. Besides, I travel with my basin. For the nutritionist, I must not soak up the pain of vomiting so as not to completely block myself from eating normally.

I am entirely dependent on Flavien. For my shower, for example, I can't stand up and if I sit down, I don't get up on my own. The other day, I crouched down to turn on the TV, I quickly found myself on my butt not being able to sit up on my own. Luckily Flavien was there and my home nurse Laurine showed us how he should pick me up properly so as not to hurt or injure me. To regain strength in my legs, I try to walk more and more every day. Barely a hundred meters, but I am improving day by day. It's a little warmer than usual this afternoon, mum is accompanying me and I almost passed out a few steps from the door. I sit up quickly and mum hands me the bucket. I want to get dressed, even though it's my only action of the day I find it makes me feel better.

During my quarantine my two millimeters of hair fell out and itchy, but I couldn't shave it. The medical team didn't want to take any chances. Too late, but I just saw a very useful solution on Instagram! As they were detached from my skull very easily, it would have been enough to stick some duct tape and by removing it from my skull the hair would have followed! This trick would have saved me days of annoyance.

A month after my autologous transplant release, while I eat exclusively sausage puff pastry, we are going four days to Île de Ré with Flavien, like last year. I borrowed a wheelchair again, the sea air makes me feel good. Then I return to the Spa de la Roche Posay with mom. I feel comfortable being bareheaded at the spa. People are used to it here, I chat with a lady who is well looked after in Tours. This summer, when my hair was just shaved, I didn't hesitate to go out without a turban, plus it was hot. But the regrowth is a fine, soft down which proves that my cut is not intentional. And my face is marked by pain so to give color I prefer to wear my shiny Entre Noue turban or my pink beret. Unlike last year, I don't have the strength to tie my scarves.

At the end of October, it has been two weeks since I vomited when I eat, and I found the time extremely long. However, I do not eat everything and in small quantities. Physical pain gave way to psychological pain. This pain makes it feel guilty because after everything I've been through I don't want my head to go down. I have no strength, I spend my days lying on the sofa. It is very difficult for me to make myself tea. It doesn't show, but it's quite an adventure when you lack the strength. After taking one of my pretty mugs from my collection, I have to open the massive drawer to choose my tea, put it in a reusable bag, then lift the heavy kettle and pour the water. And if it's empty… no tea, because it's impossible to fill it yet.

I don't want to keep getting old if it's to suffer and be dependent. I hold on to the fact that my situation is temporary, but now I understand my great-grandmother who, at 97, would sometimes tell us that it was time for her to end her life. Mémé Lydie was in a retirement home at the time and could no longer indulge her passion for reading. Still in the present moment, she had all her head to discuss. I was lucky to know her until I was 21.

Two months after receiving my transplant, it is exhausted that I see my doctor in the hospital.

- Despite a small lump that persists, there will not be a second autograft as expected. Your bone marrow is in pain.

This one-centimeter lump may not be cancerous, you can't tell because it's too deep. To consolidate the effects of the autologous transplant, I will receive antibodies, Brentuximab, every three weeks in the day hospital. And maybe radiation therapy in February, hoping for a full response afterwards. I have to take a PET scan again at the end of December. Since the treatments will be less onerous, she allows me to adopt a cat.

- But if possible not a kitten, because they are carriers of more diseases.

That's good, I want to adopt an adult in association. I don't have the strength to educate him, and many adult cats are waiting to find families. I have a fixed idea of the perfect cat and already a name, but it's been several months since I saw the photo of a tabby and white kitten. The most classic for a cat. The association describes her as fearful, talkative and fond of hugs. I see that she has been up for adoption for a year and a half ... the start of my treatments! I take that as a sign and beg Flavien to come see her. He is immediately ready and the association accepts our file. The meeting is laborious, she hides under the couch of her foster family and even the mash, which she loves, does not bring it. After a while, she heads for the kibbles, I take the opportunity to stroke her. Flavien walks over and she hisses at him. This does not prevent us, the next morning, from going to buy a litter to adopt it!

Following this inexplicable crush, we have a cat! My biggest wish, I am so happy. We rename it Kerry, as the most beautiful county in Ireland. She is fearful, but in three days she is already on the sofa with us in the evening to receive hugs on her soft belly. She's clean, quiet at night, she only scratches her tree, loves rushing up stairs, licking her teddy bear and talking… uh meow.

It's still November, but I need the Christmas magic so I'm asking Flavien for help setting everything up.

Friday 13th December, I attend a *Rose Poudrée* day. The association, of the same name, offers events between women who have or have had cancer in the Center region.

I meet Angéline and Dilek there. As a young thirty-something, Dilek reached out to me on Instagram. She lives next door to me and is also looked after in Bretonneau where we met several times. Today we have our makeup done and then photographed. There aren't many of us, but I'm intimidated to miss the target. While the others take celebrity breaks, I do the clown during my shoot. When I get home, I am frustrated that I did not take nice breaks instead of laughing out loud to hide my embarrassment. Flavien therefore suggests that I take a few photos next to the tree. They are pretty and ultimately those of the association are too. Happy with these wonderful encounters, but exhausted, it took me three days to recover.

My white blood cells are not increasing, I am still below normal. A Kopine advised me to try acupuncture and indeed in a week they tripled! I won't need to eat frozen food at Christmas.

We are reuniting with our families for Christmas, baby Léandre has a lot more hair than me! My family is small, my uncle and my aunt have taken a step back from the disease, from me. But their daughters, my two cousins, have always been there and continue to be. They are among the few people who have never made «dumplings» when writing to me. Because of the treatments, we have seen each other very little this year. So even though I'm very tired, it's nice to see everyone again. For the fourth year in a row, my Irish family sent me pajamas for Christmas. It is a tradition with them, on December 24th they receive new pajamas and spend the evening in them. It touches me very much that Sheila, the mother of a family, takes time and spends money on me.

Between Christmas and New Years, I have to have an early check-up PET scan, since the last one was inconclusive. I have sinusitis, stomach cramps and exhausted, I absolutely don't want to spend three hours in the hospital!

While waiting for the results, we celebrate Christmas, a few days after the official date, at my other grandparents. It has been a difficult night, mum advises me not to come, but I want to. It would cause me too much pain, it might be my last Christmas. After the meal and a little rest in the bedroom, I feel better, I manage to play with all my family.

But to end the year, the PET scan results are poor. The mass that was present grew and a new one appeared.

So it's never going to stop?

My parents and Flavien are present at the meeting, everyone is crying. I will receive a new treatment, I don't know which one. The Tours team must consult with specialists from a Parisian hospital. Obviously, the fear of dying is very present and also the fear of suffering with the future treatment. The autograft was so painful, I dread having to do an allograft. The principle is the same as an autologous transplant except that the marrow comes from a donor. The chance of finding a suitable donor is one in four in siblings and one in a million in the global registry. It is a cumbersome treatment and the complications once transplanted can be significant. I am not ready to go through this.

The next day, we still want to celebrate the New Year with Grégory, Flavien's cousin, and his friend Manon who has supported me a lot during the year. They are adorable and thanks to them we have a great evening. The boys cook!

For this year 2020, I prefer to focus on my creative leisure projects. Kerry manages to ease our pain. It is great to have a cat in the house. It's been barely two months and she's already very comfortable. I miss my Chanelle, who accompanied me 13 years old, but I am comparing less and less.

It's my birthday, I'm 26.
I have the hair of a newborn baby,
the concentration of a five-year-old child,
the hairiness of a ten-year-old girl,
and the inside of an eighty-year-old granny.

The antibody injection that had been postponed to January 9 ultimately did not take place. My doctor prefers that I rest all January before starting the new treatment. It is true that I have no more strength. I am exhausted.

I can't believe the results of the last PET scan. This has to be a mistake! I'm asking for another PET scan at the end of January before starting anything. It's all the fault of my head, she didn't get the message. I relaunch my research to understand the reason. I stick a post-it in my toilet with the words "I am healed", so I read it every day. And while positive thinking isn't everything, it helps me persuade myself and be more peaceful. I stop saying «my» cancer! This is not mine ! It was ONE cancer that I had, but it is no longer mine. I am breaking away from it. I educate myself on what is called spirituality. Nothing to do with religion! I have always been interested in spirituality without really putting a name on it. From a young age I was drawn to astrology with an old book that describes the signs and it amused me to read my horoscope in the newspaper. To believe in astrology is to believe in the impact of the stars on our lives ... I do not believe it, I am convinced of it! Even though it gets me a few teases and a few people trying to prove me wrong, I love to compare star signs. I noticed that some astrological signs were completely missing from those around me!

I wondered about «my why». Not «why me this is unfair», a feeling I never had, but the meaning I should give to this Hodgkin lymphoma. Since no outside factor is known for this disease, it is because I must not have understood the previous messages that my body has sent to me. The doctors take care of my physical body, I absolutely want to take care of my psychic body. Last year I wrote down the meaning of Hodgkin's disease from The Dictionary of Diseases, so on first reading it didn't speak to me, this time it was clear and logical. Blood means joy, I had lost the will to live, my confidence. We all carry cancer cells, but not everyone "triggers" cancer. I think that some life-changing event can make us sick or that if we all keep our feelings our bodies can become a pressure cooker.

We all have a different outlook on life and the world. I needed to understand and spirituality enlightened me on the meaning of life and death. So I am a soul in a physical body, but my death will only mean the disappearance of my physical body. My soul will be reincarnated in a new body and… on the way to a new karma! Although I share this theory with a lot of people, it is very personal and by no means absolute truth. This explanation comforts me in the idea of dying one day. I still have many facets of spirituality to explore. I keep some of it just for myself, because despite everything, spirituality is very stereotypical.

After an intensive month of working on my inner balance, I take the PET scan again, but despite all my efforts, it clearly shows an increase in weight.

I am therefore part of the 10% refractory to chemos1. I will be starting pembrolizumab immunotherapy treatment. Immunotherapy does not target the tumor directly, it works on the immune system to make it able to attack cancer cells by removing the checkpoints between two cells. I read on edimark.fr that «Hodgkin's lymphoma is the most sensitive cancer to anti-PD-1, with response rates in the order of 70%. These treatments could offer a definitive cure to certain patients, in particular to those in whom a complete remission is obtained».

Immunotherapy works the same way as chemo. I receive an infusion bag in the PAC over thirty minutes in the day hospital every 21 days. The side effects are few, they are mainly risks, for example the dysregulation of the digestive system or the thyroid.

Yarn to bend

French expression who mean : hard time

A few months ago, I wrote in my journal that I did not understand the lexical field of war in cancer care. Who can be this invisible enemy, if not my own body or my thoughts? Can't I fight against myself? The treatments are not a battle. Accepting treatment doesn't make me a warrior, I endure it. Won't those who don't survive cancer get beaten enough? No ! "There is no enemy when there is neither human intelligence nor intention to harm. This is a biological phenomenon that threatens us and we have encountered the test, but it is not a war ", writes, quite rightly, the philosopher Claire Marin in Le Monde. However, my opinion has changed slightly. We are fighting. We even fight all the time and for everything! To make ourselves heard by the medical team, to have rights, to raise funds for research against cancer ... As in war, we are often on the ground and yet, we get up, we suffer the lost battles, but we do not 'let's not give up!

My second injection of immunotherapy confirms that this treatment will allow me to slowly regain my strength. Apart from fatigue, I have no side effects. I am serene about the rest of the treatments, I even want to go back on escapades in France! But at the moment I am still tired and I have trouble sleeping with Flavien, I hardly fall asleep I have big chills inside my body. My two heating pads and my huge winter pyjama don't change that. I bought myself a soft and adorable Koala heating pad at the drugstore. I believe it is intended for children, but that's okay as long as it makes me happy and comforts me.

I didn't think a dream could end before it had even been realized. Since I was nine, I had dreamed of going to Australia. It's not a dream anymore, it's not even a desire anymore. Did the fear win the day or did I just get closer to the point? I no longer want to run to discover as many countries as possible. I want to take the time to discover, forge strong links with the country that makes me feel good: Ireland.

Kfighteuses
Playlist
LECTURE ALÉATOIRE
Fight song
Rachel Platten
Strong & Beautiful
Superbus
Unstoppable
Siaw
Eye of the Tiger
Survivor

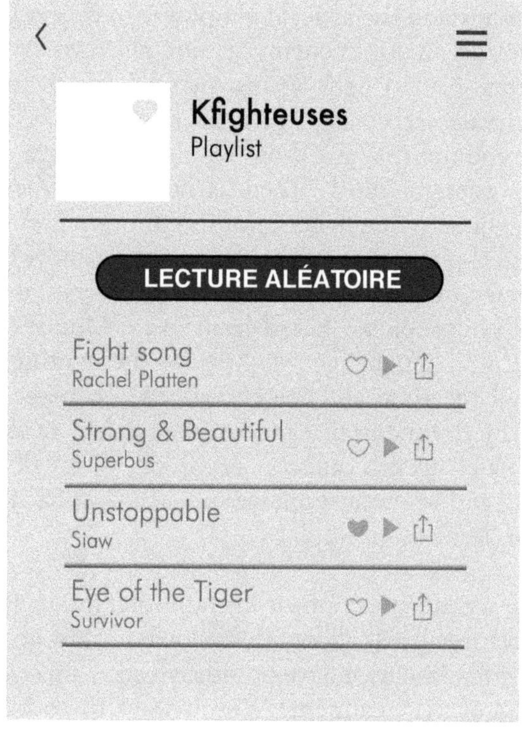

I manage to do more and more creative hobbies and this year I decided to give all my energy to the «A Daffodil Against Cancer» campaign. I offer for sale daffodil rings that I make by hand with WePAM paste! At the beginning of March, daffodils are blooming, this announces spring and is also the symbol of the fight against cancer supported by the Institut Curie and its annual campaign. Far be it from me to make any money on the back of this cause which touches me closely. For each ring sold, I donate six euros to the Institut Curie, so I have one euro left to reimburse my equipment. It all started a few weeks ago when I made myself a daffodil brooch to wear during the campaign. I then modeled a ring for my mum so she could talk about the cause at her work. It was then that I told myself that I could make more than one in order to sell them. After twelve days of campaigning, I am proud to have sold forty-two rings. This represents a total of two hundred and fifty-two euros, plus fifty-one euros in free donations. The Institut Curie will therefore receive three hundred and three euros. I am very happy with it.

During this campaign which ran from March 10 to 22, 2020, there was an upheaval in our lives. Containment! As if I had not had enough of the sterile room in September 2019! I'm used to not going out too much, we've been very careful for two years, especially with aplasia. The hydroalcoholic gel is nothing new in my purse. The only changes are that Flavien is telecommuting, so he requisitioned my studio upstairs, and my sessions with the psychologist will now be by video.

Wednesday 25th March, it is in an apocalyptic atmosphere that I go, alone, to my immunotherapy. The receptionist gives me a surgical mask, my temperature is taken twice and I rub my hands three times with hydroalcoholic gel.

With the arrival of the coronavirus, all the news channels are talking about the intensive care unit. I feel bad as soon as I see the images so I prefer to avoid them. Memories of my autograft come back to me suddenly. I can see myself again, or rather I feel again, that exhaustion, that heaviness of the body that I had felt in autograft. Two orderlies were around me, they were psychologically shaking me with the threat of going to the intensive care unit. My blood pressure was too low, I risked a coma.

- Wake up, you absolutely have to stay awake, move a little.

Everything was blurry, I wanted to sleep.

- You will not sleep if you go to intensive care because of the noise of the machines and the lights always on. Now is not the time to sleep.

I'm afraid I'll be alone in intensive care if I catch her. Even without having to be hospitalized, I just dread being sick, bedridden and not being able to do anything. So I only go out for treatment in the hospital every three weeks. And the few people who come into our house are the home nurses.

The health crisis allows me to take out my sewing machine to make a dozen fabric masks and finally learn crochet, a hobby that seems old-fashioned, but is coming back into fashion. Using videos on Instagram, I was able to make a little character from the first lessons as well as a pretty shawl. Learning something new boosts confidence, especially when I see that I am doing it and having fun doing it.

A month after the end of confinement, in June, I dare to step outside. We go to our super hairdresser, Line. A lady sticks her head through the door and asks for a place for her color. She looks at us and jokingly says:

- Be careful, because the last time a man came out bald!

She doesn't think so well, it was Line who shaved my hair last summer. I add tit for tat:

- It's crazy, the same thing happened to me here last time, I came out bald too!

The lady leaves casually. This little joke between us makes us laugh.

We resume our escapades by visiting the most beautiful villages in France near Tours. But I'm still exhausted and the months without going out haven't helped, I have difficulty walking, my legs are cotton. I lost muscle and vitality. So I rent a wheelchair through the hospital. Now after having lunch I take a nap, it is impossible to escape it. We are leaving for a weekend in Auvergne to avoid the crowds. But the fear of the coronavirus prevents us from taking advantage of our loved ones. We didn't attend Granny's 80th birthday meal or Flavien's nephews birthday.

I haven't had a PET scan since late January so in mid-August a mid-term review is in order. Immunotherapy is a long treatment, I had to wait for it to work before I got it under control. I was in the hospital for only two hours and returned three days later for the results. My doctor explains that the masses are decreasing, but there are still more. We expected the treatment to work fully or not at all. White or black. Not gray. I continue six months as planned.

A year ago, I had an autologous transplant. I'm bitter that it didn't work out and still went through all this pain.

Flavien reminds me that the pocket of the stem cells smelled like artichoke. I didn't feel anything, but everyone who entered the sterile room said so after the infusion. Perhaps this is unconsciously why I really want to eat artichoke. They say it's good for the liver! But once the artichoke is on my plate I block after a few leaves. The smell and the texture disgust me. It's not the only memory that comes back to me. I remember one evening, demoralized, singing the song «*Maman*» of Louane. In my head for hours, I even end up singing it out loud while crying. I see myself full of despair. I hurt myself so much.

«I'm not well in my head, mom.
I've lost the taste for partying, Mom.
Look how your daughter is made, mum "

Since the autologous transplant I have lost tenderness in my fingers. I am unable to touch paper, I have a constant feeling that my hands are full of dust. When I resumed embroidery in January, I no longer had the strength to pass the needle through the fabric and above all, I barely felt the needle between my fingers and the feel of the thread was not pleasant. at all. I persisted in putting on moisturizer and gradually saw progress. I'm sure the embroidery has helped me regain my sensitivity in my fingers. And what a moment of relaxation!

For the first time, I actively participated in World Bone Marrow Donor Awareness Day on September 17th on my Instagram and on my blog. It must be said that I know both sides, the donor and the recipient since I received my own transplant. I also took the two possible samples, from the bone under general anesthesia, when I had surgery on my heel bone to fill it with marrow from my hip. It's a little pain like a bruise for a few days. And a second four hour blood sample to harvest the stem cells for my autologous transplant. I did it sick and exhausted and it went well so for someone in good shape it is easy it just takes a little time. It should be noted that only 260,000 people in France are registered in the world register against 3.5 million in Germany. No, I did not forget zero in the number of French donors. Like donating blood, we talk about saving a life, except that in this situation it is even stronger! Compatibility is much lower with only a 1 in 1 million chance. In many cancers of the blood, a transplant is the one and only treatment that can save the patient. The only treatment that can keep him alive. The donor donates his time only if a match is found, the stem cells are not preserved. The donation is not made in an emergency. To become a volunteer and have the chance to save a life, simply register on the website www.dondemoelleosseuse.fr

In the hope that my period returns, I decide to stop my pill with the agreement of my hematologist. There is a good chance that I will be sterile after the many chemotherapy treatments. Impossible to have an appointment with a gynecologist who would know a minimum of the problems related to cancer treatments. The IETO37 association has recommended a gynecologist specializing in breast cancer who may be able to answer my questions. I run into the secretary who sees fit not to give me a date despite my explanations.

- Madam! You must consult a hematologist!

In the days after stopping my pill, I have hot flashes. I am certainly postmenopausal. My hormone levels were tested, but I didn't want to know the result if there was no immediate risk. However, the thyroid hormone shows an imbalance. This is one of the known risks of immunotherapy. The level is too high, a drug, Levotyrox, will help to regulate it.

While I thought my PET scan this summer was unsuitable, the medical team find it almost perfect and want to check it after nine months of treatment, not wait a year. At the beginning of November, I have another PET scan. It's early, I'm the first, but nothing is going as usual. There are new faces, the young caregiver seats me in the chair of a cubicle that closes with a half plastic curtain, right next to the nurses' office. One of them comes immediately, I can tell she's sure of her, that gives me confidence. Usually I'm in a small room and on a stretcher. So I ask him about the product. Since this is a Tep Scan that was not planned, maybe it's another product? But she tells me it's the same, but they're overwhelmed today.

I explain to him that I am difficult to sting, but precisely I did not take my blood yesterday to leave my arms intact. I have my prescription with me, she offers to fill it at the same time. It begins with the right arm.

- Do not hesitate to search for the vein, but it often happens that I have to be pricked several times. Especially in this service where the record is seven attempts. But I won't take that long!
- I won't do more than two tries, she told me before moving to the other arm.

A second nurse arrives. She wants to try again at the crease of the right elbow. I point out that I prefer to talk than to blow it works better. I ask if Marion is here today, they tell me no. Eventually she orders me to shut up and stay focused on the blood test, but this third attempt doesn't work. They want to try on the hand, but the tears rise and I categorically refuse. I'm ready to run away if they insist. It's painful on the hand, especially keeping a catheter on for over an hour when I know it's possible in the crease of the elbow! She therefore goes back to the left arm, which was already very painful from the previous attempt.

- Once the tourniquet is on, you won't feel the pain anymore, she said to me before transplanting.

This time it hurts!

- You are very very very very anxious by the bites!
- Not really.
- Oh yes, yes, yes!

After 30 minutes I suggest we wait for Marion if she arrives later.

- Marion, she's not here! We're not talking about Marion! the second nurse told me very dryly.

Back to the right arm and she starts talking to me. The first interrupts him and in a honeyed tone:

- Have you ever concentrated on a slowly flowing river?

I can't hear what she's telling me, but looking at her I realize this is the same duo that stung me seven times a year and a half ago! I am seething with rage, I did not recognize them with the masks! At the same time, the second succeeds in stinging!

- It's proven, thinking of flowing water thins the blood! And my colleague is gifted.

It's the first time I've heard this. She finally injects me with the product. I try not to think about the last 45 minutes, but I want to cry.

After an hour, she comes back to remove the infusion and adds a layer:

- When you worry it narrows the veins, the first attempt I felt the vein and when you told me about the seven attempts… Hop! She disappeared ! Next time, put numbing patches on both folds of the elbow. And on the hands! In the scanner I can't help but think of all this circus. If I am not relaxed enough, will this affect the result?

Hard prick

“ My cousin’s husband had the same than you, but he died of it. ”

Two days later, I will have the result of the PET scan during my immunotherapy. Since Monday, a new wave of interns has arrived at the hospital. After the usual questions, I ask three things internally, the renewal of my sick leave, the result of the thyroid blood test and the result of my PET scan. Ten minutes later, she returned panicked, without my stoppage of work and without my result.

- Did you see an endocrinologist? she asks me.
- No, but the blood service contacted him. How much is the rate?
- Well I know more exactly, very high… 20!
- Oh ! We're good things have gone down a lot, I was 104 three weeks ago. I am on Levothyrox. What about my PET?
- The two doctors who follow you are not here today. I started to read the report, she answers, walking away.
- Look at the bottom of the document to see if it is signed by the doctor. If it's signed by an intern, it's a temporary document, no need to read it, I'll tell him.

I am unplugged and I wait ... but after forty minutes, still nothing, I decide to go and wait in front of the office. Arriving in front of the door, they are talking about me, I stay in the half-light of the corridor.

- Oh yes, I didn't tell you, Mrs. Naudin wants a work stoppage, said the intern who came to see me.

- She can not ask her doctor? Answers a young person in a white coat.
- I don't know, this is the store here everyone has requests, she laughs, looking at the second intern.

The young man in a lab coat comes out of the office, I explain to him that I am coming for my stoppage of work and he introduces himself as a cangerologist. First time I see him, he seems to be my age. He agrees to stop me from work after asking me if my doctor can do it.

- What about my PET scan?
- Didn't we tell you? Complete remission, he announces to me as if it was the special of the day.
- But, but you tell me like that? I've been waiting two and a half years, I specify and laugh nervously.

My legs are shaky, I would have preferred to be sitting or ... I don't know what would have been better.

- Weren't you told after the autologous transplant?
- No, it didn't work. In two and a half years, the word has never been spoken.

He walks inside the office and speaks internally:

- You didn't tell him the result?
- I don't know, you are the doctor, she replies.

Well at least this intern recognizes when she doesn't know and I tell them that I prefer it to be a doctor who announces this kind of thing.

I return to the car and tell Flavien. As I explained it to him, I was filled with doubt. They've already given me a read too fast! I'm afraid this CT scan will not be as good as advertised so send an email to my referring doctor.

She calls me and confirms that the results are perfect, however, she prefers not to use the word forgiveness. I feel tremendous relief, physically it's like less weight in my chest. The immunotherapy must continue until at least February, but unlike the very first treatments I know I no longer belong in the hospital, I have other things to do elsewhere. I would definitely go back there, but to participate in workshops and meet young patients after my treatments.

The friends diagnosed in 2018 are in remission, we discuss less, because our concerns are different. I interact regularly with Lena who is one of the few people I found on Instagram with a refractory Hodgkin, for whom the autologous transplant didn't work either. She therefore underwent an allogeneic transplant and her current state of health is difficult. Also thanks to Instagram, in October, Flavien took me to Orléans to meet Fabienne who had leukemia and also an allograft, with whom I have spoken regularly for a year. Fate wanted her to come into my life, in January, when I was wondering about the connection between my body and my emotions, she is a huge help. I am also in contact with Amandine who had an autograft just before me so we are going through almost the same things. We laugh a lot by message and I hope to meet her at Le Mans soon. Talking regularly with people who understand my daily life brings me a lot.

Another indispensable Amandine, the hospital's youth nurse. Luckily she's here. She acts as an intermediary between the medical team and young patients. She takes over to explain again when you don't understand. We can confide in, she listens to us, answers our questions and reassures us. It simplifies «medical life» by relieving us of an administrative burden. For example, she synchronizes appointments so that she only comes to the hospital once a week. Psychological fatigue is important and Amandine helps me remember nothing and always makes sure that

I understand correctly. Since the start of the health crisis, she always takes the time to talk to me when I come every three weeks to a day hospital. As I have to come alone for treatment, his presence is appreciable. She shares valuable information with me, keeps me informed of events and existing associations. The first year of treatment, this position did not exist, I felt lonely as a youngster. Thanks to Amandine, I was put in contact with other young people. Before he arrived, I didn't feel so supported. I am very fortunate in having a nurse dedicated to young people. This is a real plus in the treatment process.

My PET scan from February 2021 is decisive. I don't know what they will decide for the next treatment, but I hope the results will be good. The famous Marion gives me the IV. Everything is going well. The doctor, for the very first time, offers to come and tell me the result at the end. I'm confident so I accept.

I finish my snack when the doctor arrives. We sit down and he tells me he saw something.

- I am going to examine the images, look at you from every angle and tell your hematologist about the mass on the carina.

I try to convince myself it's okay on the drive home with Flavien. I call my parents. But I crack and start to cry when I get home. My dark thoughts are coming back… I'm ruined!

Two days later, we have good news, Flavien will keep his job. With the health crisis, his company has already laid off several people. But thanks to a new project, there will be no further layoffs in his department.

That same evening, I saw the number of the blood system appear on the display. In a few seconds several questions go through my head. Shall we stop immunotherapy? Am I going for an allograft? Did they get the wrong person? My hematologist explains to me:

- The PET scan was programmed too close to the last immunotherapy. There is inflammation that we cannot take into account. I'll schedule you to have a new PET scan in a month, just before your immunotherapy.

What a relief ! Hope is allowed again. She called me not knowing that I knew about the scan results and had been waiting in complete despair for three days.

The week after, I have an ENT check-up at the hospital. At the reception, the secretary asks for my identity card. She looks at her and says to me:

- Long hair looks great on you!
- Cancer! I answer him bluntly.

I am not going to stammer and apologize for being sick. «Uh bah actually ... it's because ...» No! The reason is simple, I had cancer. His remark is not bad, I did not take it badly. I even reassured her when she apologized.

- I haven't had a bad experience with my hair loss, in the morning it's faster and I never would have dared a short haircut, this was the opportunity.

I don't think she'll dare afford that kind of comment again. I'm going to keep them a bit shorter, letting them grow out in the front for a «ball» cut.

Monday 8th March, I have an appointment at 10:45 a.m. for my PET scan, I must be fasting. Before, I will see the social worker to complete my MDPH file, because in April I will be on leave for three years. I will therefore go to invalidity. My financial aid will be considerably reduced, but for the moment I am unable to return to work, impossible to stay focused two hours in a row a day. The longer the treatments, the greater the cognitive impairment. However, I wish I could resume my profession as a multimedia graphic designer one day.

When someone has made sure that I am not too bad, they ask me if I have returned to work or if my return is being considered. The question of work also arises when I meet new people.

- What do you do in life ?
- I treat myself.

They are overwhelmed today, I go through the scanner at 1:30 pm I ask to turn on the radio during the exam. Last month, the nurse told me that all I had to do was ask, if it wasn't on. When I think back to all those PET scans in the silence, alone with my thoughts when all I had to do was ask! Last time I had Zazie's song Zen, it's funny, because I often repeat the chorus to myself for this exam.

«Had to stay zen
Let's be zen
Cold blood in the veins
Let's be zen "

This time I hear Relax from Mika! The radio sends messages to me! The exam is over, I know, there are a few minutes left, just time to go back through the machine and one last song… MY song! I loved you, I love you and I will love you from Francis Cabrel. This is the song of my baptism, it is the one I want if I get married and the one I want at my funeral. Tears always come to my eyes when I hear him. That she is passing now is bound to be a sign! A good sign. Forgiveness! I hope so.

It was only two days later, on Wednesday 10th March, during my immunotherapy treatment that the doctor came to see me:

- Two dots are still visible, but the treatment gives rise to inflammatory phenomena which can disturb the images, she explains to me.

She told me not to be alarmed when I read the report. The situation is less worrisome than it looks on paper. I am continuing Pembrolizumab for one more year.

- If I'm not in remission, what word can I use?
- What do you say about uncertain remission? she suggests to me.

I am confused. The results aren't perfect, but she seems happy and confident for the future. How long will I stay in this uncertainty? Definitely a while, because my next review will be a classic scanner in late 2021.

Three years after the diagnosis, I am still undergoing immunotherapy treatment and declared disabled. Flavien has made the concession not to return to live in the South of France, we are looking to buy a house in Touraine. I now know that we can count on each other. After only a few months together, he stayed, supported me, was 100 percent invested in our relationship. Thanks to him, a lot of things were simpler. It gives me time to regain my strength, to take a nap instead of vacuuming, to write a book instead of cooking ...

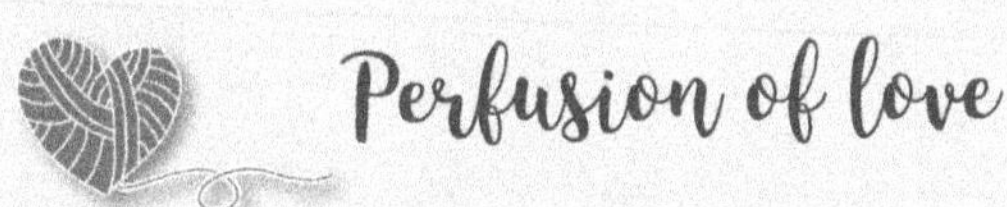

Perfusion of love

«You are strong, you are talented,
you are the one I love and nothing will be able
to change that!»

Illness robbed me of many years of carefree life and my energy. On the other hand, I bought time with friendships that maybe weren't worth it, getting to know me and what I really love. I see life differently even though I still worry so much about the little everyday problems. I don't blame my life, I sure needed cancer to grow and learn. I become legal to my family and no longer little Laura, a role in which I have enjoyed myself for a very long time. I learned to accept being seen, which was difficult for me during my first hospitalizations. It's still hard for me to say that I'm a woman and not a girl, but I'm working on it.

With this testimony, I put a big end to the face of cancer and I return to live passionately.

Forward, it's the daily renewal that carries me far.

L'avant, c'est le renouveau quotidien
qui me porte loin.

To pin

Thank you for taking the time to read my testimony. You can find me on all social networks under the nickname «Chala Moda».

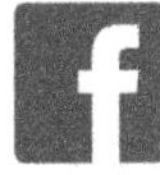 

As well as on my blog : http://chala-moda.com

To steered you

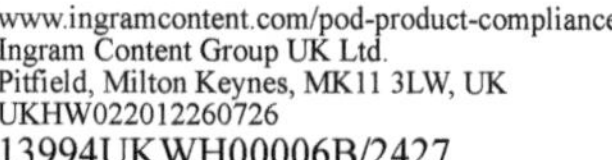

www.ingramcontent.com/pod-product-compliance
Ingram Content Group UK Ltd.
Pitfield, Milton Keynes, MK11 3LW, UK
UKHW022012260726
13994UKWH00006B/2427

9 782493 726001